So this is Kaiser

By

Frank Oliva

Dedication

My spouse – Steve Mills

My Nephrologist – Leonid Yankulin

Table of Contents

A Short History of US Healthcare

Healthcare Insurance for individuals began in certain sectors of the economy as a benefit for individuals who worked in high risk industries frequently beset by injuries, sometimes disabling, often catastrophic and also mortal.

In the 1930's President Franklin D. Roosevelt wanted to propose it at the same time he was codifying Social Security but the American Medical Association vehemently opposed it.

In the 1940's President Harry Truman tried during his administration to propose it again, but as the red-baiting of public figures like Senator Joseph McCarthy denounced anything that even hinted of socialism; he was joined by hospitals and medical associations and Truman's proposals met with the same defeat his predecessor's had met.

In 1965, part of President Lyndon Johnson's Great Society included the advent of Medicare and Medicaid to assist the elderly and poor in dealing with the rapidly rising cost of healthcare.

Since Healthcare Reform was very popular with the public many employers began to offer healthcare as an employee benefit. Unfortunately healthcare linked to employment also led to medical care "handcuffs" being placed on employees and their families. The risk of leaving or losing a job raised the prospect of losing health insurance.

Meanwhile, industrialists, like Henry J. Kaiser, realized that a healthy work force with healthy families made for a much more successful business. Henry J. Kaiser pioneered his employee healthcare system in the 1930's and 1940's. Since one of Kaiser's industrial endeavors was building the "Liberty Ships" which were an important tool in producing the Allied victory in World War II, the value of the healthcare component of his business became one of his most important assets. Other large scale employers imitated Kaiser's model. In 1945 Kaiser opened his previously private employee healthcare to the public.

President Richard Nixon, certainly no socialist or liberal, having seen the success of programs like Kaiser's and the now robust Medicare and Medicaid programs, tried to introduce his own version of universal healthcare for all Americans, but he was opposed this time from the liberal corner in the blockage by Senator Edward Kennedy who felt Nixon's proposal did not provide enough care.

So from Nixon to Obama, healthcare coverage remained a benefit for the employed, the elderly and the very poor but for those who worked for small businesses, the unemployed or those who had pre-existing medical conditions healthcare was essentially out of reach.

My Healthcare Journey

Before Kaiser

When I was born in 1952, my parents did not have health insurance, despite the fact that my father worked for an insurance company. Only 0.4% of the US population had health insurance in 1952 and my family was not part of that tiny fraction.

In those days deductibles were so high that it seemed like only the most catastrophically prone needed healthcare coverage. It was fine for those at high risk such as the men who worked in the Kaiser shipyards but otherwise it just didn't seem practical

When I, my sister and brother were born my mother had many visits to her personal physician before our births, and there were the expenses associated with the maternity hospitalization, but other than that my parents never went to the doctor. For most of the time while we lived in San Francisco I probably was the largest consumer of healthcare in my family.

The first healthcare event in my life, which I actually remember, happened shortly after my second birthday, probably in March of 1954. My whole family, father mother sister and self, were visiting my paternal grandparents. It always amazed me how noisy they and their visitors could be. They were Italian, my maternal relatives were of Irish and English ancestry and much quieter.

In the midst of the noisy conversation happening around my grandmother's kitchen table, I decided to have one of the oranges sitting on the table. Since no one was paying attention to me and my mother was holding my nine-month old sister, I picked up a knife and imitated what I had seen my grandfather doing. With my two year old hands I began to cut the orange but my lack of dexterity resulted in cutting the inside of the middle finger of my left hand.

All of a sudden, as I started bleeding profusely, everyone noticed me and immediately my father and his sister scooped me up, wrapped my tiny finger and hand in a towel and rushed me to something that no longer exists, a First Aid Station, two blocks away and kitty corner to the West Portal Tunnel. In this clinic the first aid doctor cleaned and stitched my finger and sent me home with moans and tears having survived my first medical emergency. I have no idea how much it cost but it was definitely an out-of-pocket expense because our family had no health insurance.

At age three a visit to Dr. Buckley, our family physician, had confirmed that I had tonsillitis and my tonsils would have to come out. Everything surrounding the operation was terrifying. Since my mother had to stay home with my younger sister, my father drove me to the hospital and he was nowhere as comforting as my mother. From our home in the West Portal neighborhood of San Francisco we had to drive by the dark and mysterious Laguna Honda Reservoir at night. The dark water was just one more sign of the ominous nature of this night. Why was I being driven by my father alone? Had they gotten tired of me and were they dumping me somewhere unknown?

To that point in my life I had had few interactions with strangers, so you can imagine how terrified I was of the no-nonsense very business-like nurses at St. Mary's Hospital. Then when my father left and I was all alone and a rather mean (so she seemed to me) nurse escorted me to the bathroom, I thought, "Is it possible for things to get any worse?"

I am not sure when the surgery happened. It seemed to be very early in the morning. But as if things had not been bad enough, when they wheeled me into the operating room and put something that looked like a vegetable strainer over my face to start the anesthesia, I was convinced that things could not get any worse.

On this first of my many subsequent hospital stays, I did not get to taste the notorious hospital food. My throat had to rest after surgery and I could not wait to go home.

When I got home I made sure to tell my sister that she should avoid going to the hospital no matter how bad things got. I scarred her for life and my over dramatization of my first hospital stay convinced her to stay away from doctors as much as possible. I think the only time she has been a hospital patient is for the delivery of her three children.

At three years old it is rare that one is consulted about the cost of the hospital stay but I'm pretty sure my parents simply paid the bill, we had no health insurance.

After this hospitalization I would not have any hospital stays until I became a Kaiser patient. Meanwhile, my next health care system encounter was the result of my father's intense attention to whatever might be wrong with me. When I was four, my father noticed that I had a lazy left eye. This resulted in a visit to an ophthalmologist in the historic 450 Sutter Medical Office Building in downtown San Francisco. The ophthalmologist determined that not only did I need glasses but that I would also have to begin a regimen of exercises at the University of California's San Francisco Medical Center and that my mother would have to regularly repeat these exercises at home. Both my mother and I were neither enthusiastic nor faithful in performing these exercises, much to the disappointment of the UCSF eye therapists.

After these three rather dramatic medical incidents things calmed down on the healthcare front. I don't know if was simply that these previous events cost too much for a family without insurance or what. The upshot is that it took something pretty dramatic to move my mother to take me to see the doctor. The first event happened before my brother's birth in 1960. On Good Friday, after the imposed Catholic three hours of quiet, I decided to start digging in the backyard. I don't even remember why. The result was that while digging I inadvertently dragged my palm over a shard of glass and received a terrificly deep cut in my right palm between my index and middle fingers. My mother dropped everything, wrapped my hand in a towel and rushed me and my sister into the car racing to Dr. Buckley's office on Van Ness Avenue. I went to the head of the line and my hand was cleaned and stitched and we were sent home arriving before my father returned from his office which still wasn't offering employee health insurance.

After that second hand repair my interactions with Dr. Buckley were confined to very strange wart-like painful events on my feet while I was a student at St. Brendan's Elementary School.

In 1965 a big change happened in my family's life. My father decided to change careers and become a teacher. He was offered a job at Healdsburg High School which meant that we would have to move. While I was at summer camp during the month of August the rest of my family packed everything including my stuff and moved to Santa Rosa.

Since good health insurance is usually a benefit for teachers I assume that my father got health insurance as part of his compensation package but in those days deductibles were frequently so high that health insurance was generally only used for catastrophic events whose costs well-exceeded the deductible.

During my time in Santa Rosa at St. John's and Cardinal Newman High School, I had no events that required a health care professional. Vanity had caused me to cease wearing glasses in sixth grade, so that expense was eliminated. There were two events in my brother's grammar school life which required house calls from a friendly doctor; my brother had an unusual allergy to eggs which triggered a bizarre lip swelling and he had scarlet fever, in the 19th century an almost certain death sentence. I don't think health insurance was used to pay those bills but I do not know.

When I attended Santa Clara University I actually used the infirmary when I got a terribly blistering sunburn. I was informed that there was something called student health which I guess was a form of health insurance, but I understood that if I had an actual emergency I could use this service. I didn't have to use it for anything other than the sunburn but I guess it was a form of insurance.

In 1972 and 1973 I spent my junior in Italy at Gonzaga University in Florence. I actually had two big deal medical events during my time in Europe. The first was so embarrassing, I had to use one of my professors as a translator as the doctor did not speak English and my Italian was quite rudimentary. The second was even more problematic. During the three-week Easter Break I used my Eurail pass to travel to Spain and Portugal. While traveling in the Iberian Peninsula and eating as cheaply as possible, I picked up a form of food poisoning which confined me to my bed for the last weeks of school. During this illness the school doctor visited me in my pensione room. I did not have to pay for either of these occurrences so I guess Gonzaga also had some kind of student health insurance.

After Santa Clara, I joined the Jesuits and had several small problems which required professional medical attention. I assume that an organization as big as the Jesuits had some kind of health insurance. Since I was living Jesuit poverty I had no money and I did not have to pay for any of the care I received.

Then I left the Jesuits and was on my own. I was no longer under my parents' health insurance whatever that might have been, even though I was just 22, the Obamacare coverage extending to children under the age of 26 was decades away. For six weeks I worked as a waiter which has always been an underinsured occupation. I did not have any healthcare during that period but fortunately I did not have any need of it.

In January of 1975 I began teaching at Cardinal Newman High School as a part-time employee living in the Precious Blood Rectory and I am almost certain that I was not covered by any policy. In 1977 I became a full-time lay faculty member which did include a healthcare benefit. But I was still operating in much the way my parents had. Don't use health insurance because of the deductible. Avoid doctors as much as possible unless there is no other choice.

As a young man, I had my brushes with venereal disease, and these unmentionable illnesses required, in my mind at least, a completely anonymous approach to treatment. I didn't want anyone to know about this problem and I sought a cash only transaction for diagnosis and treatment.

In 1978 I left Cardinal Newman and started graduate school at the University of California at Irvine. Before matriculating at UCI, I spent the summer in San Francisco at the American Conservatory Theater's Summer Training Congress. One of my frequent extra-curricular activities was visiting one of San Francisco's most popular Gay bathhouses, the Club Baths at 8th and Howard. On one of my visits, I met and became intimate with the man who played Mr. Peanut in San Francisco's iconic *Beach Blanket Babylon*. I became totally infatuated with Mr. Peanut, saw him at his home and then became totally obsessed. As my obsession was ballooning his hepatitis was progressing. On the night I tried to see him one more time my side pain became so acute that I had to go home, I just couldn't indulge my obsession anymore. When I woke the next morning something very strange had happened. My urine had a dark mahogany color, my feces were pure white, and the pain in my right side had escalated to unbearable. I did not know it at the time, but I found out that these three symptoms were classic signs of hepatitis.

In July of 1978 I had no insurance and no job. I had to struggle to get to the University of California at San

Francisco Medical Center. In those days they were still treating the indigent for free. I was seen and diagnosed but then was told that the only treatment available was rest, complete rest. Since I was planning to start graduate school in September, this unexpected medical crisis almost derailed my post graduate plans. Well, I healed quickly enough to drive to UCI in time for the start of school.

UCI definitely had student health insurance and student dental care and I used them both. Most of the events that required professional medical care were relatively benign: colds, sprains, nothing very dramatic until my 28th birthday.

My housemates thought it would be fun to celebrate my birthday with a roller-skating party. Skating around Newport Beach Harbor on a warm and beautiful February 23rd seemed like a great idea until I took an unexpected fall which was not particularly surprising considering my lack of coordination. The fall resulted in a lot of pain but no broken bones and a lot of embarrassment.

Once I had received my MFA in stage direction from UCI, my student healthcare came to an end. The good news was that I got a job immediately out of grad school with San Francisco Opera as a production assistant. The bad news was that because it was technically a part time job and one without a union affiliation, it did not qualify me for health insurance. This status was to last from 1980 until 1987.

During my years at San Francisco Opera my rather promiscuous behavior led to many infections with venereal disease. I had so many visits to the San Francisco Venereal Disease Clinic that they had to tear up my visit card several times. The good news was that despite the shame of visiting this clinic, it actually was not so bad. In fact it was very cruisy place and I sometimes met future sex partners including one of the doctors who treated me.

One memorable moment in my health care journey happened on a beautiful Saturday morning in June of 1981. I had gone running early that morning and as I returned to my Upper Market apartment I passed the kiosk outside of the then Star Pharmacy (now Walgreens) at the corner of 18th and Castro. Typically the entire *San Francisco Chronicle* was posted on this kiosk and one of the front page stories was about a newly discovered "Gay cancer."

I thought, "How ridiculous. Now we even have our own cancer." I was bemused but not worried. I should have been, this was the first time hearing that the disease that would eventually be labeled Acquired Immune Deficiency Syndrome, or the acronym AIDS, was printed in a newspaper.

My frequent visits to the VD Clinic continued, then in mid-1982 I played with a friend who unbeknownst to me had genital herpes. He left me with that gift. Once again without insurance I had no immediate recourse to medical care. I don't know why I didn't go to UCSF or the VD Clinic, but I didn't. I guess I just didn't think I could afford the necessary medicines.

But this discovery scared me a lot. All of a sudden it became clear that my promiscuous behavior was also very dangerous.

There was a phrase for those who had not been identified with the immune compromised men who were dying in droves but were more than likely candidates for future diagnosis; it was the "worried well." I was definitely worried and I began to change my behavior.

One thing that happened because of my new worriedness was a referral to a therapist. I had an appointment before I had to travel to the East Coast, but the interruption meant we would not meet in earnest until September. Meanwhile, I was a little more circumspect about my sexual behavior but not much. At his suggestion I started to keep a journal.

While I was keeping the journal, my drinking, which I would never describe as moderate, accelerated. I found myself more and more out of control. By November my therapist was encouraging me to investigate sobriety programs. Throughout this period I had no insurance and could not pay for therapy, but my therapist, realizing how much I needed it, did not end my counseling.

For the next three months my behavior got worse, my visits to the VD clinic increased and my periods of drunkenness became more frequent. During that period I experienced something I had never before experienced, protozoan infection of the bowel. Despite the fact that I had no insurance; the clinic doctor prescribed the horrible drug Flagyl. It seemed worse than the symptoms for which I was taking the drug.

All of these physical problems led to the worst Christmas I had yet experience. I was so sick; I had to eat rice while everyone else was having prime rib with all the trimmings. Coupled with my therapeutic experiences I was quite miserable.

Finally, in March 1983, my therapist decided he could no longer treat my problems without assistance. He mandated my membership in a program fostering sobriety. With this mandate, my life took a 180^0 turn. I started abstaining from alcohol and drugs and I actually stopped having sex with anyone.

About six months after this 180^0 shift, I received an unexpected phone call from one of my former sex partners. He had called me from Sloane-Kettering Hospital in New York. He had called me to tell me that he was one of many Gay men who had been diagnosed with what was called at that time in New York City, GRIDS, Gay Related Immune Deficiency Syndrome; what would eventually be labelled as Acquired Immune Deficiency Syndrome, AIDS. He was in Sloane-Kettering being treated for pneumocystis pneumonia.

This was a real wake-up call. After the initial scare which led me to therapy I gradually became less frightened and in my sexual abstinence felt as though I had dodged a bullet. The call changed everything. I learned that not only did San Francisco have the free Venereal Disease Clinic way down on Fourth Street across from what would eventually become Moscone Center, it also had neighborhood health centers which were also free. The closest to me was Health Center 1, on 17th just east of the Castro.

Sheepishly I went to Health Center 1 as a drop in patient. I related my ominous phone call to the triage nurse who was not particularly shocked by my story. He treated me with kindness and quickly placed me in a room with one of the doctors on staff. The doctor took my medical history, paying particular attention to the tale of the phone call from my former sex partner who had called me from Sloane Kettering.

In 1983, GRIDS or AIDS was so new that no one had any idea how the disease was transmitted. Some speculated that it was a new sexually transmitted disease like syphilis or gonorrhea, perhaps it was transmitted like the amoebic dysentery from which I had been suffering in late 1982, and there were even those who speculated that it was caused by the use of amyl nitrate, a sex enhancing inhalant that increased the intensity of orgasms by stimulating the pleasure centers of the brain. But in 1983 there were no definitive markers. So the way doctors tried to determine who was infected was by a kind of circling the wagons technique. They looked for other related sexually transmitted conditions such as chlamydia to see if that might be an identifier.

The first sign that this mysterious new illness might have some common denominator was when they found that children and hemophiliacs with no excessive or abnormal or homosexual history also were detected with the illness, then researchers began to look at the blood supply and a transfusion history that might indicate that this illness was passed by blood and not necessarily by sex.

Up until this point I was unable to hold or keep a full time job and in those days, before the Affordable Care Act, only the independently wealthy could afford private health insurance, and most employee health benefits were only offered in companies with a large number of employees, and those benefits were rarely offered before a probationary period.

In January 1984 I got a job with a very small sign company and there were no health insurance benefits before or after a probationary period. Small businesses simply could not afford the premiums associated with employee health insurance, so my small business never offered me this benefit. Still, since I now had full-time employment, despite the minimum wage I was receiving, my therapist expressed his expectation of payment now that I had a little more cash.

By the summer I had started to work at an insurance company, but once again the probationary period prevented me from receiving health insurance. I almost made it to the end of my probationary period, before I quit for what I thought would be a better job. It wasn't and I found myself back on the street, unemployed and uninsured again.

During this time I was still in therapy and without insurance, only able to pay a small fraction of the amount my therapist normally charged per session. Meanwhile, with each passing day I lost more and more friends and acquaintances. I would see someone at a meeting or on the street, and the next week I would read in the *Bay Area Reporter,* the newspaper of the Gay Community, of his sudden death.

I went from the "worried well" to a member of the "totally freaked out Gay Community." In spite of the horrible headlines, after almost a year and a half of total sexual abstinence I returned to a very active and somewhat dangerous sex life. With regard to sex I was a lot like what Talleyrand said about the Bourbon monarchs, I had "learned nothing and forgotten nothing." I started to date a lot of guys as I was continuing my therapy. My therapist didn't react in horror or scold me. He just encouraged me to be safe and careful.

In 1984 and 1985, two events drove home the frightening closeness of AIDS. One night after a meeting a friend came home with me, he wanted to show me something.

Not thinking it was a big deal, I thought, "Why not?" He raised his pant leg and revealed a small raised black dot. He told me it was his first Kaposi Sarcoma scar. I was horrified. Then about six months later at one cousin's wedding, a Gay cousin, who was less than two years older than me, told me that he too had Kaposi Sarcoma.

After a lot of disappointing halfhearted short relationships, I met Steve Mills at an ATM near Ralph K. Davies Hospital. I fell for him at once and we started dating. Steve had health insurance and a very good job. I was still trying to balance a fledging opera stage directing career with intermittent temp jobs, and I still had no health insurance. Steve moved into my small one bedroom apartment a little after a year of dating me.

During that year of dating a major breakthrough had happened with regard to AIDS. Researchers had been able to identify an anti-retrovirus in the blood that caused a drop in the T-cells. Because the presence of the antibodies associated with this anti-retrovirus could jeopardize one's health insurance, the city had begun offering anonymous blood testing to determine if one had or did not have the antibodies. It would tell a patient if he was positive or negative. With trepidation, Steve and I went for our tests on a beautiful Saturday morning in February of 1987. We would not know the results for two weeks. They were not the most delightful weeks we had spent.

I was not terribly surprised when my results came back positive. I guess Steve was, because he went into a terrible depression which eventually resulted in a serious hospitalization. Along with his depression over his positive status, he was fighting another serious illness, Crohn's Disease. The perforation in his large intestine was slowly bleeding him dry. Steve' poorly treated Crohn's disease was not properly treated until man years later, but finally was remedied by surgery.

Meanwhile I started to have difficulty breathing. I went back to Health Center 1 where I had first been studied for a possible infection that would eventually be called AIDS, and where Steve and I had taken the blood test which in 1987 was termed HTLV. The Health Center 1 doctor suggested that I seek testing at UCSF as they did not have the funds or the facility to do it themselves.

I went to UCSF seeking the tests and found out that they would do them for this "worried well" patient, but that since I had income and no insurance, the testing would cost me over $300.00 of my own money. The results of the tests, which included a very painful arterial blood draw, determined that I really had nothing wrong with me aside from testing positive for the virus that could result in AIDS.

I call this episode the "financial cure." While Steve was suffering from severe depression, I had had enough. I stopped worrying and determined to get on with my life.

In March of 1987 I had one last opera directing assignment before I changed from being a temporary employee to be a full-time employee with an insurance company. When the last temp job turned into a regular full-time position with health insurance, being not very rich, I chose the cheapest plan offered to me, Kaiser's.

My Healthcare Journey

With Kaiser

Chapter 1

Kaiser Before My Catastrophe

I directed my last professional opera at Sacramento Opera in March of 1987 and then returned to San Francisco to continue working at Industrial Indemnity Insurance Company, but no longer as a temp, now as a full-time employee with health insurance. It began a journey that continues to this day. It was and is the first time I was and am part of an HMO, a health maintenance organization. I had had student health insurance, high deductible health insurance as a teacher, and no insurance for the period from graduate school graduation in June of 1980 until March 1987.

With hopeful eyes, I began to discover what "this is Kaiser" meant and means. In 1987 I was relatively healthy and dismissed my urgent need for health insurance. Like everyone else I had the occasional cold. The colds usually followed the family celebrations of Thanksgiving and Christmas and the interaction with the germ machines otherwise known as school age nieces and nephews.

When I felt too sick to go to work, I girded my loins and headed to Kaiser hoping that I would not have wait an hour or more to see the doctor who had been assigned to me with no prior consultation about the compatibility between us. Usually the results were very disappointing and it convinced me that I better be a lot sicker before I made that trek and wasted that hour or hours, only to end up disappointed as I headed for work.

I don't remember a lot of blood testing during this initial phase of my relationship with Kaiser. Sometimes on the respiratory infection trips there would be a throat swap to see if I had strep throat but that was pretty much it.

One unusual experience was a period in my relationship with Steve where we both realized that we were having trouble communicating. We sought couples counseling but we were both somewhat disappointed in the results. Whether it was Kaiser's fault or ours, I'm still not totally certain, but the good news is, Steve and I are still together, in fact we got married in 2008.

Life with Kaiser continued without much fanfare until my schedule changed. After about a year at Industrial Indemnity, during which time I was trained in the programming language, Nomad, a friend at Bank of America recruited me to become a Nomad programmer in the Consumer Credit Division.

When I changed jobs and got a very nice raise I had to go on COBRA to continue my Kaiser insurance. Of course I had to pay for the COBRA because at this point in my health journey I could no longer coast without health insurance and since I had already had a year with Kaiser health insurance Kaiser was the cheapest option for me, even as expensive as the COBRA was I really had no other choice. In 1987 I had tested positive as an immune suppressed Gay man. Without health insurance I would be in a very dangerous territory. However at this point I was still only HIV-positive. I still had a primary care doctor who seemed homophobic to me and who I really did not like but there didn't seem to be any other alternative.

Chapter 2

Kaiser And My Catastrophe

After eighteen months in which I had been working in a satellite office building on Montgomery Street in San Francisco there was a reorganization of the Consumer Marketing Division. This reorganization resulted in our programming section of this division being relocated to Concord's huge Information Technology campus known by the acronym BASE which stood for Bank of America System Engineering.

Our safe little programing group was now part of the big behemoth. It was somewhat intimidating. This move had a major effect on my commute. Since most of us were San Francisco residents this relocation resulted in an exponentially longer commute. The good news was that the Concord BART station was just across the street from the BASE campus. The bad news was that there was a fifteen minute interval between trains to and from Concord. It was not unusual for me to intend to leave my desk allowing me time to walk the significant distance from my IT building to the BART tracks only to see that train that I had been anticipating taking, charge out of the station as I entered the turnstile which then required me to wait another fifteen minutes for the next departing train. Since I usually worked until 5:30 PM and sometimes past 6 PM I rarely arrived home before 7:30 PM which made dinner a very late meal.

After four months of this schedule I started to feel extremely exhausted on a regular basis, in fact daily. In 1990 the unfortunate reputation that Kaiser had garnered in relation to persons with immune suppression, even those who had opportunistic infections which were related to immune deficiency, was not good. Through the Gay grapevine I learned that the only reliable Kaiser doctor who was effectively treating Gay men with immune deficiency was Stanley Hill and his very capable Nurse Practitioner, Pat Saunders. With my new malaise I decided to change my primary care physician. I elected to be a new patient of Dr. Stanley Hill.

In the twinkling of an eye everything about my health care changed. Suddenly I was having regular appointments with Dr. Hill and sometimes Pat Saunders. In fact, an index of my wellness corresponded to which medical professional I was seeing. If I was doing OK, it was Pat, if not so good, it was Dr. Hill. The other thing that happened is that I started to have many more blood tests at a much greater frequency. Although testing T-cell counts had been used to help diagnose immune deficiency in the early days of the AIDS epidemic, I had never had a T-cell or CD4 count until I began to be followed by Dr. Hill. The first count done around April or May of 1990 was terrifying with the result of 228. Normal is in a range from 500 to 1000. I had a count significantly lower than the lowest number of the so-called normal range.

The way that medical professionals were and still are using the T-cell counts was and is as a guide to investigate which opportunistic infections could possibly affect their patients. For patients with numbers like mine, the doctors were testing for the opportunistic infection, pneumocystis carinii pneumonia (PCP), which in 1990 insured almost certain death. One medication that could seemingly prevent PCP was aerosolized pentamidine. Intravenous pentamidine was the last resort when the pneumonia was already in full flower.

In these early days of the AIDS epidemic the indifference of the Reagan administration with regard to the wholesale destruction of Gay men caused a delay in medications that would try to address this epidemic. Meanwhile, underground un-FDA approved medications were being distributed by neighborhood clinics like the Lyon-Martin Women's Clinic. Since Kaiser would not distribute any drug which did not have FDA approval, my doctor and nurse practitioner suggested that I might want to investigate these clinics without actually their prescribing them. Steve and I went to the Castro Area clinic as each experimental medication appeared. First was un-approved AZT. Then came DDI, then D4T.

The bad news is that none of these medications appeared to have any positive effects and AZT had many harmful side effects. The friend who had assisted me in getting my job at Bank of America succumbed to the deadly side effects of AZT when he died in January 1991.

In 1990 after eight months of a lengthy BART commute from San Francisco to Concord and back plus the malaise I was experiencing from my weakness due to my falling T-cells I finally reached a breaking point in early August and a profound disagreement with my boss caused me to seek a new programmer position with Bank of America in San Francisco.

As I was starting my new position as the programmer for the Secondary Marketing Division of Bank of America, Steve, having survived his depression over his HIV positive status, now faced a more immediately daunting health problem, aggressive Krohn's disease. The large intestine wound caused by the Krohn's disease was leading him to experience significant anemia. Normally robust and ruddy the anemia was making him appear as white as a sheet. Fortunately, he had very good health insurance but the prognosis was not good.

I continued to see Dr. Hill and Nurse Practitioner Saunders and didn't experience a lot of problems. Because I was so vulnerable to pneumocystis the physicians tried to get me to take dapsome, a prophylactic medicine against the pneumonia, but it had a serious sun sensitivity component, and I was quite averse to avoiding sun exposure so of course I got the predicted body rash. They next prescribed aerosolized pentamidine. It was a very obnoxious therapy involving hour-long boring weekly inhalant sessions.

In January 1992 I had my first big scare. It was no longer just fear of something happening. This time something did happen. Perhaps it was precipitated by all the fear coupled with the stress around Steve's illnesses but what happened is that I began to feel a strange tingling on my right back and sides. I had no idea what it was, it was just something very uncomfortable which I had never experienced before.

My Auntie Flo was a regular attendee at the San Francisco Ballet and since we had regularly been attending the opera for several years, including a couple of opening nights, she asked me to join her for the white tie Ballet Gala Opening. I actually had a set of tails and the requisite white tie of which I did not have many opportunities to use. Little did I know that while attending this Gala with a firm starched white tie shirt the itching that I had been feeling would flare up into a full blown case of shingles. The performance was unendurable but I said nothing.

When I got home I checked and sure enough the tingling side and back had blossomed into a line of purpled bumps stretching from my back to my belly button. The next day I was able to see Nurse Saunders who confirmed that I indeed did have shingles and she put me on a very strong course of Acyclovir. She explained that any child who had had chicken pox was a candidate for shingles and that frequently the condition was triggered by stress, as I had had from my worries about Steve and my own diminishing immunity.

In 1992 Steve and I began taking the drug D4T, it seemed to be one more useless anti-retroviral therapy. Shortly I was to find that this drug had many unfortunate side effects.

As lifelong Democrats, Steve and I had become exhausted by twelve years of Republican presidents and we had actively campaigned for Bill Clinton. We not only contributed money but we actually engaged in active politicking, we joined the hosts of phone banks at the California Nurses Association and made cold calls to Democratic voters urging them to get to the polls.

When Bill Clinton squeaked into a victory with a plurality instead of a majority against his opponents, sitting President George H. W. Bush and independent Ross Perot, we immediately decided that we wanted to participate in the celebration. We wanted to go to Washington to attend Bill Clinton's inauguration.

Living in the bluest of blue congressional districts we were unable to secure inauguration tickets from our congresswoman, Nancy Pelosi, so we sought tickets from a very Republican Congressman. I had a relationship with workers in the office which "shipped" the loans we had sold in the Secondary Market. That office was in Orange County and one of my contacts in Orange County suggested that perhaps her newly elected Congressman, a Republican, could secure tickets for me and Steve.

Having secured our tickets, we both requested a week's vacation for the week surrounding the January 20th Inauguration Day and made the rest of the necessary travel arrangements. Throughout the Thanksgiving and Christmas Holidays we could think of nothing else.

We flew to Washington on the Monday morning preceding January 20th and thoroughly enjoyed the Democratic Celebration occurring in DC. We visited virtually every historic site and museum along with the White House, Congress and Ford's Theatre.

Washington was particularly cold and clear in the penultimate week of January 1993. One of the more spectacular events was the celebration in front of the Lincoln Memorial of the official arrival of the Clintons and the Gores. Unfortunately, for events of this kind the celebrities arrived much later than they were expected. While we waited we decided to sit on the very cold ground of the Washington Mall. Though there was no snow, the ground felt like the permafrost of the Siberian tundra.

We had an incredible week in Washington during the Clinton Inauguration. Once returned to San Francisco I tried to resume my usual mile-a-day swim at the YMCA. But what used to be invigorating turned into an impossible endeavor. After only one lap I was so out of breath that I had to get out of the pool. The next day I made an appointment with my Nurse Practitioner who on consultation with my primary care physician, presumptively diagnosed me with congestive heart failure with pulmonary edema. A chest x-ray confirmed their diagnosis, and so for the first time I was placed on medical leave from my job for three weeks and placed on Lasix to eliminate the edema, the fluid in my lungs.

Dr. Hill ascribed my new medical condition as a reaction to the experimental anti-retroviral I had been taking, D4T. It wasn't my first opportunistic infection but it was certainly a warning as had been my shingles episode. If I had been frightened before I now was officially scared.

Chapter 3

Waiting for the Big One

After the D4T congestive heart failure and pulmonary edema episode of late January and February of 1993, I was seen more frequently by Dr. Hill and Nurse Saunders. They started me on Dapsome cautioning me to stay out of the sun. Their caution went in one ear and out the other.

While all this was happening to me, one of my best friends, Mike, was having his own set of nightmares. Mike was about seven years older than I. He had been married, been in the Viet Nam war and had a much harder time developing a long term partnership with another man than I did. We both found out about our HIV infection about the same time. He had had various unusual infections, which I had not had. One very unfortunate thing that he did that jeopardized his prospects of going onto the Social Security Disability Insurance, that might have extended his life, is that earlier in his life he had fraudulently collected those benefits and so to be able to begin collecting them now that he needed them he would have to repay the fraudulently received money. His financial position was such that he was absolutely unable to repay the money hence he could not get the benefits he now desperately needed.

Watching him go through this process was particularly painful. He had become such a dear friend to Steve and me but we felt helpless facing his dilemma.

Throughout the spring and early summer Mike got worse and worse. When a fellow college alumnus of his was to be ordained to the priesthood for the San Francisco

Archdiocese in April, Mike asked me to drive him. He was so incredibly weak; I had to help him in and out of the car.

As April slid into May, Mike was declining faster and faster. So were many of our other friends. What was happening to me is that although I had no more health scares like the congestive heart failure or the shingles, I had sworn off any anti-retroviral. When Steve and I went to our family vacation home in the Sierra, even though I was taking dapsome, I did not avoid solar exposure and so I got the expected rash, all over my body. Dr. Hill and Nurse Saunders decided to place me on aerosolized pentamidine therapy in lieu of the dapsome. Several times a week I had to take time off from work for the late afternoon therapy. I didn't care that much, I had pretty much lost interest in work.

Steve and I had had such a great time when we went to Europe in 1991 that we decided to do it again. Despite the fact that we had already used up one week of vacation time for Bill Clinton's Inauguration, we thought we could spend another three weeks traveling in England, France, and Italy.

One of the Europe experts in Mike's travel agency planned a splendid trip for us. Meanwhile Mike was fast approaching death. In despair over the denial of the lifesaving SSDI benefits, Mike went to his doctor and asked for an easy way to get out of life. Assisted suicide was not legal in California in 1993. In fact it just recently did become available, but Mike got him to prescribe a hospice style exit, an accelerated morphine drip that began on June 25th and by the night of June 28th it had done its work.

June 1993 was a very hard month for me and Steve. In addition to Mike, we had lost my very good friend, Gary, Steve's former lover Michael, and a mutual friend of me and Mike. We were extremely depressed but these losses had become so common that we had lost at least one friend or two a month for the past eight years. Still we were fully intent on making our European trip.

During the month of July, after Mike's funeral, my T-cells were falling faster and faster. My medical team was of the opinion that I should stop working. Despite the lack of enthusiasm and energy I had about my job I was in enough denial that I refused to recognize the physical and mental stress I was experiencing. I did not want to go on disability no matter how bad my performance at work was.

After trying to convince me it was time to stop working, Nurse Saunders decided to refer me to a therapist who worked in the Member Services Department. I actually was not clear about why I was being referred to him. His name was Jerry and he definitely seemed interested in helping me. I just couldn't figure out why. I tried to tell him what a vital resource I was for Bank of America's Secondary Marketing Department.

Over the past several months I had been having night sweats which were often the first symptoms of pneumocystis pneumonia, but I had tried to ignore them. I told Dr. Hill, Nurse Saunders, and Jerry about the night sweats but in the same breath I tried to dismiss them.

Jerry encouraged me to go to Bank of America's Human Resources Department to find out what my options might be regarding disability. The good news was that since I had joined Secondary Marketing I had been paying $7.00 a month for Long Term Disability Insurance. What this meant is that once I started drawing Social Security Disability Insurance and my State Disability Insurance expired after a year I would draw the equivalent of 60% of my current salary until I died or reached the age of 65. So financially, things would not be as bad as if I had stopped working with no benefits.

Still, I was not ready to go on disability and I still wanted to take the European vacation with Steve. At our last appointment in August, before Steve and I left for London, Jerry and I decided we would continue this discussion when Steve and I returned from Europe in early October.

Steve and I left for London two weeks after Labor Day. We flew from London to Paris and then flew to Milan. We spent several days in Florence where I started to have more night sweats. One late afternoon in Florence, on the street running from the Duomo to the Ponte Vecchio, I sat down on a step and started crying. I had finally accepted that I was very sick and would probably never see my favorite city again, the place where I had spent my magical junior year of college, and to which I had made so many other incredible visits. Then we visited my relatives in a small city near Salerno. During the Salerno visit we spent several days on Capri and that's where I really started to have a major problem with breathing and night sweats. By the time we got back to Paris and London I could tell that I was getting very sick. We arrived back in San Francisco and I knew I had to see my doctor or nurse immediately and contact my counselor Jerry.

Chapter 4

Pneumocystis – the First Opportunistic Infection

On the morning of October 3, 1993, having safely returned from what I thought would be our last European vacation; I went to Kaiser to see my medical team. I recounted my difficulties breathing while in Europe and the recurrent night sweats. I was presumptively diagnosed with pneumocystis carinii pneumonia, pending the results of the x-rays and blood tests which had been ordered.

Before we left for Europe I had numerous conversations with Jerry, my counsellor, regarding the possibility of going on disability and my reticence to do so. With the presumptive diagnosis and a recognized disabling opportunistic infection (colloquially referred to as OI's) , the ball was no longer in my court.

I went to work and immediately saw my boss. She wanted to accompany me for my conversation with Human Resources. Both Linda, my boss, and the woman from Human Resources were incredibly compassionate, helpful and consoling. We agreed that I would officially go on disability on October 15th at which point my Secondary Marketing Department would throw me a going away party, something between a retirement party and a wake.

In 1993, a diagnosis of pneumocystis pneumonia, an AIDS qualifying opportunistic infection, was nothing short of a death sentence. My last day at Bank of America was extremely sad for me. Having finally found a job at which I was excelling, going on disability felt like a loss of identity. I was only 41 and 65 was very far in the future, a future that I felt I would unlikely see.

I guess my medical team did not think I was that sick. Instead of putting me on the very caustic drug IV-pentamidine, they prescribed an oral medicine called clindamycin. I had started this drug on the day of my presumptive diagnosis.

Once I had gone on disability on October 15th, I had to see the disability counsellor at the Social Security Administration to become eligible for the Social Security Disability Insurance and receive California's State Disability Insurance. When State Disability would end after a year, it would be replaced by the Long Term Disability Insurance to which I had contributed when I started working for Bank of America's Secondary Marketing Division. What an incredibly lucky choice I had made.

So far everything had seemed very easy. Everyone lined up to make this an almost seamless process. The one thing that wasn't being addressed was my sense of despair. After all, in 1993 an AIDS diagnosis was still a death sentence. There were some medications that tried to address the more severe consequences of the opportunistic infections, but nothing had succeeded in stopping the deaths.

After a month on clindamycin things were not going well. Not only had the drug not changed my pneumocystis infection I had developed a severe allergy to it which had similar allergic effects on me as had penicillin and dapsome, any solar exposure resulted in a severe rash. My doctor decided that I would have to take a much stronger medicine. In 1993 the only alternative to oral medication for this severe form of pneumocystis pneumonia was intravenously administered pentamidine. I had taken the prophylactically administered aerosolized pentamidine, but that was before I had the full blown disease. Now, after a month of ineffective oral medication I was going to start treatment in the Kaiser Infusion Center.

In 1993, the Kaiser Infusion Center was not in the hospital, or a clinic in a medical building, as it is today. It was in an old converted store front occupying a small corner of the current San Francisco site where the main medical building of San Francisco's Kaiser main campus stands. If you weren't aware of it you would never have noticed it. I had never noticed it. I had never even been on that side of the street.

By that time it was the beginning of November. I had wasted October taking an ineffective drug. My pneumocystis infection had become much more virulent. I went to the Infusion Center with a greater amount of trepidation than I had when I saw my medical team after our European trip.

On the first day of infusion I was greeted with friendly faces, a lot of paper work and an ominous back room to the store front filled with chairs that looked like recliners surrounded by IV poles.

Every one of the nurses greeted me as I was assigned a chair of my own. The nurse assigned to me invited me to sit in the recliner and then asked me in which arm I would like to have my infusion needle inserted. If I had told the truth, I would have said neither, I hated being stuck for blood work and this seemed much worse. Since I had been born with a right-handed dominance, I offered my left arm.

Being infused with anything, including saline, is awful. Being infused with pentamidine is a lot worse. It burns. Not only that, this treatment requires daily infusions for three weeks if one can survive it.

It was during the first week that I realized I would need more help than just my infrequent visits with Jerry in Kaiser's Member Services. I was a member of Most Holy Redeemer Parish in San Francisco's Castro District. I started seeing Sr. Theresa, the Pastoral Associate of that parish.

Being seen by Sr. Theresa was a life changing experience. She wasn't a part of my bodily health care team provided by Kaiser, but she did make some incredibly powerful suggestions which changed my spirituality. She was a member of the religious sisters of the Blessed Virgin Mary, more commonly known as the B.V.M.'s. The B.V.M.'s were not only associated with Most Holy Redeemer Parish through Sr. Theresa's presence, they had also been the order which staffed Most Holy Redeemer School until it closed in the 1970's.

Sr. Theresa recognized that my relationship with God was clouded by a great deal of fear. She proposed that I adopt the concept of a "Grandma God." A God who loved me in the way my maternal grandmother had loved me – totally and unconditionally. It resulted in a complete 180° turn. Gradually I morphed from having a very angry judgmental image of God to one as loving as my late grandmother Marjorie and I think this change allowed me to move from extreme fear to hope.

Another change that happened in November, while I was having daily infusions of the very caustic pentamidine, was joining a group sponsored by the Most Holy Redeemer AIDS Support Group. With eight other guys and wonderful facilitators I began to share my pain and fear with my peers who were experiencing the same things I was.

Even though I had been told I had an AIDS defining deadly opportunistic infection, I still had great difficulty admitting that I actually had AIDS. Thank God for the nurses and the other AIDS clients in Kaiser's Infusion Center providing a joyful comradery equivalent to the survivors on the *Titanic*.

The Infusion Center was not restricted to AIDS patients though we were definitely the majority in the mid-1990s. Sometimes there would be patients who required a blood transfusion but they usually were appalled or disgusted by our devil-may-care attitude, not to mention their disdain for us obviously Gay patients.

One of the things about a three week course of pentamidine infusion is that it starts out painfully enough – it took sometimes two or three stabs before the nurse assigned to me got the IV needle into the vein in which they were going to infuse, but then it got way worse.

As the treatment progressed into the second week, the systemic effect of the pentamidine caused increasing weakness. Having pneumocystis provides its own concomitant challenges, labored breathing due to the infection in the lungs plus the expected rise in white blood cells due to the presence of a deadly infection take their toll. But as the infused drug is attempting to kill the deadly infection it starts interfering with the other important bodily functions. One of the most deadly effects is its attack on the digestive system.

Halfway through the second week, my appetite was disappearing. By the beginning of the third week I had completely lost any desire to eat. One night Steve presented me with a dish of my favorite pasta, penne with red sauce. With no appetite and a body filled with poison I refused the meal. I had even lost the ability to swallow even water. In a fit of frustration and pique, Steve grabbed the plate of pasta and flushed it down the toilet and immediately followed that with his own dinner saying, "If you're not going to eat, I'm not going to eat."

During this period of infusion and malaise, I spent most of the time, when I was not going to the Infusion Center and being infused or returning home, lying on the couch watching television. One of the worst experiences was watching an early dramatization of Tony Kushner's AIDS epic, *Angels in America*. Early in the play the character with a full blown AIDS diagnosis is forsaken by his lover who cannot face the trauma of caring for an AIDS patient. Aside from my fear of my death sentence this was my next greatest fear.

One of the wonderful things that happened during my daily visits to the Infusion Center was meeting Nurse Iris Perris and getting to know her and appreciate her passionate care for all of us stricken with opportunistic infections made possible by the AIDS virus, which required daily or twice daily drug infusion. As my three week course neared its end and I became incredibly weak, the nurses started talking about the reward I would receive if I completed my treatment. In fact when one of the patients who had started his treatment a few days before me completed his treatment the nurses brought out a little motorized figure of a hula dancer. With the celebratory mood of a birthday party, they switched on the hula dancer and amidst much laughing and hilarity the hula girl did her dance which almost brought us all to tears.

My turn came a few days later and I was tremendously grateful as my IV was withdrawn after twenty-one days of torture. The required treatment had been completed and all we needed to do was find out if my blood tests would show that the pneumocystis infection was out of my system.

By this point Thanksgiving was just a few days away and I had many reasons to be grateful. I had survived my treatment. Steve had survived my treatment. I had been cared for by amazingly compassionate Kaiser nurses, and I felt that my appetite was returning.

The first two pneumocystis pneumonia experiences were amazingly eye-opening. I learned that knowing about AIDS and hearing about AIDS was nothing like experiencing the opportunistic infections to which it subjects the patients.

The coming Christmas season was relatively uneventful, a kind of lull before the storm. I continued to see Dr. Hill and Nurse Practitioner Saunders, Counselor Jerry and Sr. Theresa. I was fully engaged in the MHR AIDS Support Group, deriving a great deal of information and identification. Up until this point I had had a very difficult time identifying myself as an AIDS patient, very similar to my unwillingness to identify as a Gay man. Once I started to feel better I even decided to resume my exercise routine.

I was by no means well after this autumn of challenge but it seemed I was no longer in as bad shape as I had been as our European vacation was ending. One bit of bad news related to the European vacation which I hadn't anticipated suddenly raised its ugly head. Since Steve and I had taken a week's vacation to attend the Clinton Inauguration and our trip to Europe had lasted three weeks, I thought I had used the four weeks that had been guaranteed me. But, those four weeks had been predicated on twelve full months of work. Since I officially went on permanent disability on October 15th, my employment did not include a full year and therefore my vacation time was in deficit. This affected my State Disability Claim and hit me with a financial penalty for which I was not able to pay. Fortunately, my own beloved former boss was able to intervene and I ended up not losing any income, but I did lose a couple of nights of sleep.

Not much happened until my birthday approached in late February 1994. I began having the typical night sweats and breathing problems associated with the onset of pneumocystis. A visit to my physician and the concomitant blood tests and x-rays confirmed my suspicions. I was embarking on my third episode of pneumocystis and of course the requisite visits to the Infusion Center.

This time I knew the drill. The personnel in the Infusion Center were no longer strangers; in fact they had become very compassionate care givers. Despite the ordeal I knew I would have to endure, I was very glad to see them again. The first time I went to the Infusion Center I was relatively unaware of the other opportunistic infections treated with infusions. While I was there I had met many who were being infused for Cytomegalovirus Retinopathy, abbreviated CMV. In fact, my good friend Walter Fernandes had been infused for both pneumocystis and CMV. I don't remember as much about the second infusion period as the first, but I know it had the same devastating effects.

When the second infusion of pentamidine ended my weight had gone down as well as my T-cells. But I was ready to return to the gym, and then one night in April 1994 I awakened with extraordinary pain in my side. I immediately asked Steve to drive me to the Emergency Room at Kaiser.

Because of my severe pain, I quickly jumped whatever line preceded me. After a number of stat tests and discussion I was presumptively diagnosed with a kidney issue and I was infused with a drug which caused hot flashes and made me very uncomfortable. The good news is that the drug relieved my pain, the bad news was yet to be revealed.

Chapter 5

Diabetes

After my third bout of pneumocystis and my second pentamidine infusion I was exhausted. I needed a break. And even with that mindset in April, I experienced the kidney emergency which fortunately was relieved by another drug administered intravenously.

Just as I thought I might return to a life resembling disability normal, something totally unexpected, at least to me, happened. I started experiencing sudden weight loss and fatigue. These were not symptoms of a recurring incidence of pneumocystis but they did necessitate another visit to the Emergency Room.

When I got there I was put into a special room, my blood was drawn and tested stat. Steve, on returning from work had found me in this distressed state, before we could even contemplate dinner. While I waited for the blood work, Steve went to one of our favorite Noe Valley Italian restaurants and returned with one of their delicious entrees.

Meanwhile, when the ER doctor returned with the test results, he announced that my blood sugar had revealed that I was a diabetic. This diagnosis "floored" me and also angered me greatly. I had been avoiding sugar in my diet for the previous eleven years. This diagnosis hurt my pride. I had become a passionate zealot on the issue of sugar as poison. This simply was a diagnosis I could not understand.

Diabetes has never been identified as an AIDS opportunistic infection, but in my case it essentially was. It required me to seek explanations and discover the many changes that would be required in this new dispensation. I was given a dose of insulin in the ER and then sent home with an appointment with my own doctor and with the endocrinologist who supervised Kaiser San Francisco's diabetic patients.

My diagnosis did not leave me in a good mood. Since my primary medical crisis was AIDS, diabetes was treated like an unwanted child. I already had a death sentence so diabetes did not seem to be a big deal to me or to my physicians.

At my first appointment with my Certified Diabetic Educator I learned the protocols of administering insulin and may or may not have been instructed in blood glucose testing, but from this vantage point all I remember is that I was told to inject myself with a certain amount of long-acting insulin thirty minutes before my first meal of the day.

At first the whole routine regarding diabetic care exhausted me. Perhaps it was my anger regarding becoming a diabetic after being so cautious around the consumption of sugar for the previous eleven years. I resented the fact that I had become a diabetic.

My first response was to jettison my no sugar diet. I began to consume sugar with reckless abandon. But as the insulin I was taking every morning began to help me regain the weight I had lost during my pentamidine treatments and the subsequent onset of diabetes I started to have more energy which allowed me to begin doing a lot more exercise. I began biking everywhere except where it was necessary to drive. I resumed my exercise routine at the YMCA.

During my first visits to Dr. Hill and Nurse Saunders, it was explained to me that one of the things that pentamidine could do while preventing me from dying of pneumocystis pneumonia was that it could also destroy my pancreas. The kidney pain Emergency Room visit had been simply a wakeup call warning me and my medical team that there was something much graver happening.

Something unusual happened around the same time all the diabetes problems were happening. Whether she had initiated the process before or after I went on disability, my boss, Linda, had submitted my name for a departmental Bank of America EPAP, which stands for Exceptional Performance Award Program. To be perfectly honest, from the time I had gone on short term disability after the Clinton Inauguration to the two weeks return to work after our European vacation, my performance had been anything but exceptional, it had been downright abysmal.

Nevertheless, Linda had recommended me for the monetary award and someone had approved it. At the beginning of May 1994, about the same time as my diabetes diagnosis, I received the unexpected check. It was enough money for Steve and me to take a trip. As a way to thank him for his exceptional care during my three bouts of pneumocystis and the kidney and diabetes episodes, I decided I would take him to Las Vegas as a thank you gift.

We booked several days in a Las Vegas hotel, reservations on a prop plane tour over the Grand Canyon and great seats at Cirque de Soleil's *Mystere,* the first time we had ever seen that amazing troupe. But the most startling thing that happened is that I began to eat regular deserts from the menu. Steve had never seen me do this before and he was horrified.

Despite the new complication of diabetes joining the other difficulties I had been having since my definitive AIDS diagnosis, things were going remarkably well all things considered. But learning how to manage my diabetes was more complicated than I thought.

Still, I was putting on much of the weight I'd lost during the several pneumocystis bouts of the fall, winter and spring and by summertime I was biking almost every day to the YMCA and swimming while I was there. I was doing so well that Steve and I decided to take a Hawaiian vacation.

When we went to Hawaii in 1992 we intended to visit two islands, Maui and Kauai. The night before we left Hurricane Iniki did massive damage on the big island and practically obliterated Kauai. Maui itself sustained significant damage, including the beach in front of the hotel where we had reservations. Since the hurricane happened less than twelve hours before our flight, there was no time to advise us that our plans might have to be changed.

Once we arrived at our hotel bits of information began to dribble in and by the following day it had become clear to us that Kauai would no longer be our second island. We had a lot of scrambling to do with regard to both our second hotel and the way we could fly home.

Because we had missed Kauai in 1992 we decided to try again in 1994 because of the recovery I had made over the past year. One of the biggest attractions in Kauai is the rugged beauty of the Na-pali coast. A trail wide enough for animals as small and nimble as mountain goats runs along sheer cliffs over one hundred feet above the Pacific Ocean. This trail was at the top of our must see and hike list. The first point at which the trail met the ocean was purported to be approximately one half hour's hike into the trail. We decided that that would be a good point to turn around. Unfortunately we had not considered taking some form of carbohydrate with us in case the excess activity lowered my blood sugar. I was still a novice in the use of insulin and I never considered how it and exercise could lower my blood sugar.

As we returned back to the trailhead I began to behave very strangely. On the narrow goat trail high above the

Pacific I started to walk erratically getting dangerously close to the cliff edge. Steve, fortunately, was able to guide me to a safer trail away from the cliff and get me to sit down. But my blood sugar was falling and Steve was stuck with the dilemma of leaving me by myself in order to get something I could eat, or staying with me and watching my blood sugar fall.

As if sent by Heaven, two men rounded the curve behind us and asked what was wrong. Steve explained that I had diabetes and was having a very low blood sugar. Miraculously, the two men who had rounded the curve behind us were doctors and one of them was a pediatrician specializing in diabetic children and not only that, he had a power bar which he was willing to give me. Like manna from heaven his power bar was consumed by me. We had faced and been delivered from our first diabetic hypoglycemic nightmare. We promised ourselves that we would never take that risk again, at least we hoped not.

We returned home having enjoyed and survived our Hawaiian vacation. Deep in our minds was the fact that the year before I had been a ticking time bomb as my pneumocystis infection was approaching explosion which would become the identifying opportunistic infection to officially certify me as an AIDS patient.

With my new regime of insulin and exercise I was a lot healthier than I had been the previous year. Unfortunately my T-cells were not as robust as my outward appearance. Despite the falling T-cells and my diagnosis as an AIDS patient who happened to also be a diabetic, my aggressive biking and exercise routine rendered me no longer insulin dependent. I had been freed from the regular blood testing and insulin shots. I was very happy about this progress.

Chapter 6

Cytomegalovirus Retinitis

The man who ran the Most Holy Redeemer AIDS Support Team that sponsored the support group which I continued to attend weekly, informed me that his partner like my friend Walter was so debilitated by CMV Retinitis (a disease caused by a micro-organism called Cytomegalovirus which attacks the retina in one or more of the eyes finally causing blindness and more frequently than not in 1994, death), was very close to death.

In 1994 the typical treatment was an infusion more caustic than that used for pneumocystis. I first encountered patients receiving it during my several pentamidine infusions. While the pentamidine course was once a day for three weeks, the CMV retinitis infusion had to be done twice a day and for a much longer period. I learned that from my friend Walter. He had been infused for pneumocystis the year before I was, had then had the CMV retinitis infusion.

The difference between the persons who got pneumocystis and those who became CMV retinitis patients was the value of the T-cell count. When my count was in the 200 range I developed pneumocystis. As my T-cells approached 100 I became much more susceptible to CMV retinitis.

As I had been frightened about being diagnosed with AIDS before it happened, I began to fear any of the myriad opportunistic infections that were lying in wait for me as my T-cells continued to plummet.

There still are many trials for drugs addressing both AIDS and its accompanying opportunistic infections. In 1993 most of the drugs were either in development or in their infancy. Those of us who were already identified as infected with HIV or designated as AIDS patients with opportunistic infections intrepidly sought studies which were both remunerative and potentially life-saving.

I had heard of a UCSF study of a drug which might be useful in the treatment of CMV retinitis. I had not been identified as a CMV infected patient but my T-cell count was low enough to qualify me for the study. I had made the necessary applications but had not heard from any UCSF personnel.

In September of 1994, while Steve and I were vacationing in Kauai, I retrieved a voice-mail from Brooke Anderson, who then served as the study coordinator for the safety and efficacy portion for a CMV retinitis drug. When I called her I learned that I was a perfect study subject and that participation would involve two full days of hospitalization and pay a gratuity of $500.00.

I was very excited about participating in the study and receiving the rather large gratuity. After we returned to San Francisco from Hawaii I was scheduled to be a study patient in November.

The study was tedious and as far as I know the drug that was being tested never made it past the FDA and into the treatment formulary to treat CMV retinitis. Nevertheless it was my first participation in an AIDS Opportunistic Infection drug study.

Over the course of the next year my T-cells continued to fall and I had other opportunistic infections which will be discussed in later chapters. Throughout the course of 1995 my problem with my eyes had not been diagnosed but my problem with almost daily diarrhea was becoming more acute.

As the almost certain approach of my death seemed more imminent, Steve and I began a program of what became monthly travel. We started 1995 with a driving trip to Hearst Castle in January. We flew to Las Vegas and drove to Death Valley in February. In April we went to Honolulu to visit some San Francisco friends and then flew to Maui. We took other short trips around California including King's Canyon and San Diego.

We had become good friends with the UCSF study coordinator, Brooke Anderson, and through her had learned about the Franciscan mission near Santa Fe mentioned in Willa Cather's novel *Death Comes for the Archbishop*.

When I read Willa Cather's masterpiece, especially the part about the mission at Chimayo, nicknamed the American Lourdes, we decided that we had to go to New Mexico in August. Steve and I flew to Albuquerque and drove to Santa Fe intending to see the mission and the operas at Santa Fe. We also were able to visit the archbishop's ranch in the suburbs, do whitewater rafting on the Rio Grande and spend some private time in the sacristy of the Chimayo Mission. Steve anointed me with the "sacred dirt" from the sacristy floor.

Despite the many high points of our Santa Fe trip, it was very hard on me. One of the other opportunistic infections that was plaguing me was a form of wasting manifested in incredible diarrhea. This outrageous diarrhea would ultimately be the cause of placing me on morphine and in hospice, but that was still lay a year away.

On our flight back to San Francisco, our layover in Denver resulted in something completely unexpected. Because of the extreme August heat and the higher than usual demand for seats on our flight, United Airlines offered any passengers willing to take a later flight, a voucher of $750.00 per passenger. Up until that point Steve and I had had no plans for another major trip in 1995. We had been to Hawaii and Santa Fe, but the unexpected vouchers allowed us to plan another big trip. We decided to fly to London and then travel by Chunnel to Paris in October.

In November, our friend John Marshall invited us to visit him in Palm Springs. This was our last monthly trip of 1995. During the course of this year my vision problems had become more challenging. My fear was that the specter of CMV retinitis that was haunting me now seemed to be manifesting with the increase of annoying floaters, something of which I was previously unaware, nor had experienced. The first "sighting" occurred when I began to see small black dots clouding my vision, they looked like tiny bugs. They scared me enough to ask my doctor for a referral to ophthalmology. I was seen several times by what seemed to me to be a junior ophthalmologist, but when, in December, he noted the radical increase in the floaters, I was dilated and sent to the ophthalmology photographer. The drop in my t-cell count had also alerted my entire medical team that I was now a prime candidate for a CMV retinitis infection.

After the very painful series of photographs were reviewed I was promoted to the care of the senior ophthalmologist, Dr. Wolitz. I was very glad about coming under his care as he came highly recommended by my friend Walter. Dr. Wolitz discovered that the damage to my right eye's retina was significant enough to order me to begin infusion. It had been almost eighteen months since my last pentamidine infusion and something unexpected, at least by me, happened.

Kaiser San Francisco had finally gotten the approval to build a brand new medical building. Since my last pentamidine infusion in April 1994, construction of the new center had begun and one of the buildings destroyed to make way for the new center was the old store front which had housed the Infusion Center. The new temporary Infusion Center was on the second floor of the Walgreens on O'Farrell Street, across the street from the old medical center.

When I arrived at the Infusion Center, I was greeted once again by my friend and infusion nurse, Iris, from my days as a pentamidine infusion patient in late 1993. What was different this time, was that instead of the once a day infusion of pentamidine that lasted for three weeks, CMV retinitis required twice a day infusion of ganciclovir until the infection was eradicated. Another difference was that since the Infusion Center had a normal eight hour a day schedule, the center would not be able to infuse me twice a day. The only solution was to start me with an IV in the Infusion Center in the morning and then send me home with the bags of drug and an IV pole, so I could infuse myself.

However, there was one problem that no one expected; I was allergic to the latex of the IV. When I arrived at the center on the first day of infusion things followed the typical pattern. I was seated in the infusion chair, the IV was inserted in my vein, and the drug was infused. I went home with a very uncomfortable IV in my arm, but I was ready to try it that night. The IV became increasingly painful throughout the day up to the hour when the infusion needed to happen that evening.

With resignation, Steve hung the bag of liquid drug and attempted to flush my IV line. Nothing happened. As much force as he applied to the syringe it wouldn't budge. It was too late to contact anyone in the Infusion Center and the pain in the infusion site had become so intense that there was only one solution. Steve had to remove the

IV, abort the infusion and wait until the following morning before we could return to the Infusion Center and start the whole process once again.

With embarrassed grins, we arrived at the Infusion Center only to be met with hostile disappointment. It felt like they were blaming us for the failure. The actual villain was my allergic veins, but they were not convinced. They reinserted the IV in a new vein, infused me, sent us home and hoped that I would be able to infuse that night.

Unfortunately the same thing happened again and I missed another dose of medicine. We actually tried once again, but with this failure everyone threw in the towel punting me back to Dr. Wolitz.

He had a solution. In lieu of the twice daily infusions he substituted pills, many many pills. With the pills in tow I returned home only to have another set of photographs and an appointment with Dr. Wolitz to determine the state of growth of the lesion and the decline of the vision in the infected eye. The bad news was that the drug in pill form was not being as successful as the IV drug was purported to be.

After several weeks of pills Dr. Wolitz decided to change strategies. A new protocol had been developed for patients like me. But it was much more gruesome than its predecessor. It was much like the old child's oath "Cross my heart and hope to die. Stick a needle in my eye." Dr.

Wolitz told me that he would have to give me intra-ocular injections once a week.

I was horrified. I simply could not imagine this procedure. Nevertheless, the CMV retinitis disease having not been able to be addressed by normal treatment had progressed and now required desperate action to prevent complete vision loss.

Having recognized the clear and dire straits we had reached, Dr. Wolitz told me we had to do the first treatment that day. He prepared the syringe with the liquid ganciclovir, placed a speculum around my right eye which would keep me from blinking or flinching, placed some sort of numbing medicine in my eye, had me turn away from him, and surreptitiously wielded the syringe plunging the needle into my right eye.

There actually was no feeling but I experienced an audible and extraordinary pop, louder than a pin piercing an egg or a balloon. It caused no pain but the psychological jolt was tremendous. And I would have to experience this weekly trauma for the foreseeable future.

While Dr. Wolitz was treating my CMV retinitis, the issue of CMV being able to attack my other eye in the absence of a full body treatment haunted me and him. Injecting the right eye only affected my right eye. So when an untested drug purported to address the systemic issue of CMV infection became available, he suggested that I become a research subject. In addition to the regular and frightening intra-ocular injections, I would have to take many more pills and have the painful dilation photographs every week along with my injections. This would last until the effective drug cocktail that would reverse so many AIDS deaths became available.

My relationship with Dr. Wolitz continued until his much lamented retirement in 2012. He was a wonderful and caring ophthalmologist and I miss his care and friendship very much.

Chapter 7

Dermatology

And Dr. Goldstein

AIDS is a tremendously complex combination of illnesses and diseases. Its name, Acquired Immune Deficiency Syndrome itself, defined as a group of symptoms that consistently occur together or a condition characterized by a set of associated symptoms, is more complicated than a simple disease like diabetes. Syndrome indicates that it embraces many diseases caused by the collapse of the immune system. This collapse, triggered by an anti-retrovirus infects immune suppressing T-cells. The anti-retrovirus has been named human immunodeficiency virus, a virus named for its activity, opens the patient to many opportunistic infections.

My own experience was no different. The AIDS defining infection for me was the onset of pneumocystis pneumonia which was identified positively in October 1993. As a result of the treatment to prevent that disease from killing me, the drug used ended up destroying my pancreas and making me a diabetic. AIDS involves many hard choices and many slippery slopes.

Before AIDS caused these very big problems, I had skin problems. Several of the drugs that had been prescribed for me caused rashes as one of their possible side effects. If there was a possible side effect, no matter how minimal, I usually got it. So, once I received Kaiser Insurance it wasn't long before I was referred to Dermatology.

More often than not, I was disappointed with the dermatologists who saw me. They were either dismissive or not very interested in my dermatological problems and often gave me very little care beyond prescribing some kind of cream or lotion and sending me on my way.

But once I was diagnosed with AIDS the dermatological care changed. Some of the providers didn't want to have anything to do with me. Since one of the other more common opportunistic AIDS defining diseases was a skin cancer called Kaposi Sarcoma, dermatologists seemed to expect AIDS diagnosed patients seeking their services to be potential KS patients, but one of the ironies of the AIDS complex is that usually those diagnosed with pneumocystis rarely got Kaposi Sarcoma and vice-versa.

Probably because Kaposi Sarcoma was such a heartbreaking disease with few solutions if any, dermatologists were reticent about enthusiastically treating AIDS patients.

The bad news for me was that as my opportunistic diseases were increasing in numbers, my T-cells were falling, and my health was becoming more fragile and the envelope that encased me, my skin, was also being traumatized, as was the rest of my body.

I don't remember the first time I saw Dr. Goldstein. I just remember complaining to one of my fellow Most Holy Redeemer AIDS Support Group members, (Walter) that I could not find a dermatologist who responded to my needs or addressed my problems. Walter told me that he had started being seen by a new dermatologist, Dr. Goldstein. He was very pleased with the way he was being treated by him and suggested that I ask to be seen by him.

I was so relieved to hear this that I made an appointment with him as soon as possible. Dr. Goldstein was so different from the others that I had seen. He seemed genuinely interested and genuinely concerned.

I honestly don't remember why I needed to see him in the first place. It might have been a rash or a drug reaction. I know that the sun damage my scalp had experienced from many years of unprotected sun tanning and sun burning was becoming a severe problem. I had this terrible nervous habit of continually scratching a point on my scalp. And, unfortunately, there were a lot more than one spot. Whether, it was caused by nerves, infection or actinic keratosis (pre-cancerous sun damage) I simply would not stop.

Dr. Goldstein, instead of dismissing me and my problems, showed me that he was willing to work with me to try and find the causes, the effects, and perhaps the cures necessary.

Unfortunately, he and I were facing the unstoppable drop in my T-cells and my collapsing immune system. In spite of the amazing odds he was facing, he never gave up. He was always scrambling for the next answer.

As my situation became more and more hopeless he did some amazing work. One of his solutions was to refer me to another dermatologist at UCSF. He was not afraid to look for other solutions, even if they didn't come directly from him.

I remember being sent to a strange clinic out in the shopping center that use to be called GETS in the Avenues on Sloat Boulevard. I had to go to an office at UCSF. Every dermatologist I saw outside of Kaiser threw up his hands in dismay.

At this point there was no solution for my constantly itching scalp. Everything that was tried did not work.

Meanwhile as my T-cells were plummeting to the point where I had become vulnerable to CMV Retinitis, and even lower when a particular form of tuberculosis also termed an opportunistic infection made possible by the immune deficiency caused by AIDS, was accompanied by a new opportunistic infection directly affecting my skin. This so-called new to me opportunistic infection was called molluscum contagiousum. This annoying endstage disease manifests whereby the very exhausted immune system allows tiny microorganisms to populate all over the body and face appearing as miniscule red dots.

The only way to remove these microorganisms is by the brutal almost barbaric process called curetting. In simple terms, Dr. Goldstein took something that looked like a infinitesimally small melon baller and bloodily melon balled my body and face until I no longer could bear it.

When Steve and I lived on Eureka Street, during this point in my AIDS journey, we had a friend three doors away, named Richard Sparks, who frequently greeted me on my way home from Kaiser. On each of these occasions he asked, "To what indignities has Kaiser subjected you today?" We would laugh and I then briefly would describe the "melon balling" as his face contorted and he writhed in pain.

This process did not end my relationship with Dr. Goldstein, there would be many other visits in which we dealt with the skin problems caused by my weakened immune system and the problems caused by the medications prescribed to me, but at this point I need to discuss other aspects of my care at Kaiser.

Chapter 8

The Opportunistic

Infections

As I've said before, AIDS is a very complicated medical syndrome. What it does by lowering the immune system is open the body to infections which would normally be controlled by a healthy immune system.

Again, it's the reason why doctors treating AIDS patients keep such a laser focus on the T-cell count. The count is an indicator to prepare doctors for which opportunistic infections they may expect to find based on the count.

I had been described by Dr. Hill and Nurse Sanders as a "refusenik." After my bad experience with D4T in 1993 I was unwilling to try any of the new treatments that were coming on the market, approved or in trial. The first protease inhibitors had made their debut in 1995. A number of members of my Most Holy Redeemer AIDS Support Group were actually in trials of the new drugs. But I was maintaining my "refusenik" status. The new drugs seemed just as risky as the D4T.

But while my situation was moving from grave to bleak I continued to stand my ground. And the bleakness was being revealed in things like aggressive diarrhea, and increasing weight loss (at one point my weight got down from 150 pounds to 95 pounds), the drugs had caused so much difficulty with bowel movements that I had to see the surgeon, Dr. Stricker, for such horrible anal problems.

But the extreme weight loss which accompanied the T-cell drop prompted Dr. Hill to test me for a type of AIDS related tuberculosis acronymed MAC which stands for

Macro Avium Complex. I am not sure what the relationship with the avium, birds, is, but it was a very nasty disease treated with an equally nasty drug. Perhaps it was the MAC that prompted my extreme weight loss but the acknowledgement of my weight loss led to a diagnosis of wasting. Both of these situations contributed to my extreme diarrhea, which sometimes resulted in twenty bowel movements a day.

When one looks at the AIDS quilt, there is one fact that cannot be dismissed. If one were to use the quilt as a graph of the devastation wrought by AIDS, one would be struck by the extreme drop off in deaths after 1995. Unfortunately the numbers did not remain low, but the advent of the protease inhibitors and the AIDS "cocktails" did provide a startling halt in the previous years' cataclysmic deaths. But in 1995 I was still a "refusenik." I was not willing to risk the potential side effects, I had had enough from the necessary drugs I had to take and the anti-viral medications I had taken prior to diagnosis had done nothing.

My friend Walter, who was in the MHR AIDS Support Group, and I were constantly joking about the idea of getting the equivalent of a Boy Scout merit badge for each diagnosed opportunistic infection. But the reality was, they were taking their toll on my psyche and causing an acceleration deteriorating health.

As the opportunistic infections mounted, my health care team started to scramble. It seemed that while all these opportunistic infections were potentially lethal the one that seemed to alarm the team more than others was the wasting.

You never know where the solution arises, but when you are desperate you pay attention to those who hold out a ray of hope. Dr. Wolitz, my ophthalmologist had a very kind nurse. This nurse also worked with the AIDS research department at Kaiser. At one of my appointments with Dr. Wolitz, she told me about some experimental success that was being seen in using Thalidomide with AIDS patients with extreme wasting. She felt that this might work for me and she arranged for me to see Dr. Fessel, the Kaiser doctor running the study.

First of all, I must mention that there was a lot of fear around Thalidomide. This once hyped drug was used to assist women in the late 1950s with nausea and morning sickness related to pregnancy. The tragedies resulting from the use of this drug were the infants whose mothers took this anti-nausea medication and were born with undeveloped limbs, arms and legs much shorter than properly formed children.

Once the relationship between Thalidomide and these horrifying birth defects was verified the drug was retired and regarded as poison, but desperate AIDS researchers in looking for anything that might help with the multitude of debilitating conditions AIDS was causing in those patients who did not die from the primary opportunistic infections looked to Thalidomide as a possible remedy.

The Kaiser AIDS research department had started trials on drugs like the resurrected Thalidomide and these researchers decided that I would qualify as a candidate who might benefit from taking this previously frightening drug, but naturally I was skeptical. Obviously, since I am male there was no prospect of fetal birth defects, but the unknown was still frightening. Nevertheless, while facing my rapidly declining weight and being cajoled to try something that might work, I decided to participate in this study.

By this point in my AIDS journey, accompanied by the wonderful caregivers of Kaiser San Francisco I had succumbed to the following opportunistic infections: Pneumocystis Pneumonia, Cytomegalovirus Retinitis, Macro Avium Complex, AIDS relate Tuberculosis and Wasting; but they were other non-opportunistic problems and they will be discussed in the next chapter.

Chapter 9

Jerry Geffner –

The Psychological Component of AIDS

I mentioned Jerry Geffner in one of the first chapters when discussing my journey at Kaiser around my own AIDS crisis. I was sent to see Jerry by Pat Saunders, Dr. Hill's nurse practitioner, because both she and Dr. Hill knew I needed to stop working and go on disability, and they also knew that it would be a particularly hard sell to me despite my weakened condition, they needed a more convincing advocate and they chose Jerry Geffner.

Jerry Geffner, who holds a Master's Degree in Psychological Counseling, in 1993 was working in Kaiser's Member Services Department with the assignment to assist those diagnosed with AIDS, 90% of whom were Gay men, with the transition from a working member of society to the loss of income due to disability and the services that might be available to them.

As recounted in an earlier chapter, my acquaintance with Jerry began in August 1993. His first task was to convince me that my health was not good enough to allow me to continue working. At first I refused to buy his reasoning. I was in a great deal of denial about this issue. After a number of sessions he persuaded me to consider the issues we had discussed. Since Steve and I were embarking on a three week trip to Europe in early September, we decided to postpone these decisions until we had returned from Europe.

During our travels in England, France and Italy my health deteriorated progressively. On several nights in our hotel in Capri I experienced night sweats which drenched me and my sheets. Our hotel on Capri had an Olympic sized swimming pool which I found irresistible. But when I attempted to do several laps in this pool I experienced the same shortness of breath which I had experienced when I was diagnosed with congestive heart failure in February. It seemed that the handwriting on the wall was clear. The decision I was unwilling to make before we flew to London was now immanent. I recognized that my time was up.

When we arrived back in San Francisco, I had two appointments, one with my doctor who immediately sent me for blood tests to confirm what he suspected: that I had pneumocystis pneumonia; the other appointment was with my Member Services counselor, Jerry Geffner.

The blood tests and x-rays confirmed that I had pneumocystis pneumonia and therefore AIDS. The meeting with Jerry Geffner was to continue the discussion which we had left in suspense when Steve and I flew to Europe. But after the events in Capri and the presumptive diagnosis the discussion took a very different turn. Before Europe I had been very reluctant to even entertain the thought of going on disability for AIDS. After the trip and subsequent diagnosis I no longer had any hesitation.

Jerry and I decided that I would inform my department head of my decision, give her a two week notice, consult with Human Resources to learn my options, and leave my employment at Bank of America on October 15, 1993. Despite these decisions, I still was ambivalent.

In 1993 an AIDS diagnosis was still a death sentence. Virtually every single person who had been diagnosed with AIDS had a two year life expectancy. This was not the trajectory I wanted. An AIDS diagnosis was almost always accompanied with many problems other than medical issues. The biggest was the confusion and depression caused by the immediate realization that a normal life expectancy could no longer be *expected*. And that's when Jerry Geffner began to play a much more important role in my life and mental health.

Jerry had been such an incredible help in my early days with AIDS that I had to be grateful for whatever help he might give me. For most AIDS patients, once Jerry had guided them through the red tape of disability, Social Security and the prospect of having to deal with the malaise and lack of activity resulting from the side effects of illnesses and the cessation of regular employment that preceded disability, his time with the patient was concluded.

Perhaps, because I had had so much difficulty with the decision to even go on disability or actually accept the fact that I had been diagnosed with AIDS, Jerry decided that I needed help beyond the complex process of making sure Kaiser patients diagnosed with AIDS had all the resources available to them, even the ones with which they were unfamiliar.

Ending my career at Bank of America was psychologically wrenching. Although my body was absolutely screaming to be put on disability, my mind was still saying "No!" It took the diagnosis of pneumocystis pneumonia to push me into disability. And Jerry realized that it was just the beginning of my psychological trauma.

Once the first hurdle was crossed and I stopped working at Bank of America on October 15, 1993, I was left with a very confusing life. Suddenly I had nothing but time on my hands. I needed the kind counseling Jerry offered me. He may have exceeded the normal boundaries of his office, but he regularly made time for me.

By November it had become clear that the first treatment of the disease had failed. Instead of arresting the progress of the disease, the drug had caused a miserable rash and left me in worse shape than on the day of diagnosis, Because of this I was forced into the next lifesaving process, IV pentamidine infusion.

The daily sessions in the Infusion Center made it even more clear that I needed Jerry's counseling. Additionally at this time I sought spiritual direction from Sr. Theresa, B.V.M., the Associate Pastor of Most Holy Redeemer Catholic Church, and I joined a men's support group offered by Most Holy Redeemer's AIDS Support Services.

Jerry continued to see me about every two or three weeks and we became very good friends. Seeing Jerry was an opportunity to recount the difficulties I was experiencing with the various side effects from the treatments that I was receiving. Also, I had the opportunity to discuss the sinking feelings I was having related to not working.

Throughout my life I have had a problem with anger. With the gradual acceptance of my AIDS situation, the anger reaction was going from a low simmer to occasional full boils. As pneumocystis infections went from second episode followed shortly by the onset of diabetes, full boils were occurring much more frequently than low simmers.

The increasing frequency with which these anger flare-ups were happening was becoming a major problem. On one of the many occasions I had to drive to Kaiser either for a medical appointment or a psychology appointment or a treatment, the rage I was feeling went out of control when something like a skateboarder cutting me off while I was driving occurred.

Then it happened, I tried to cross Market Street at Castro on a very ripe yellow light because I was late for my appointment with my long-suffering therapist, Jerry Geffner. Actually the light was yellower than I thought and a police cruiser witnessed my red light running. I was stopped, ticketed and had an emotional breakdown. I made it about two-thirds of the way and that ticket had put me over the edge. I pulled over in tears and called Jerry. He suggested that I have someone come to where I was parked and drive me to my appointment.

During the appointment Jerry and I came to the conclusion that it was time for me to hand over the car keys. I was no longer deemed to be safe behind the wheel and my driving privileges were revoked in the late summer of 1995.

By November of 1995, just before my treatment for CMV Retinitis, I had another major breakdown. Something had happened that upset me so much that I couldn't stop sobbing and couldn't get out of my rocking chair. Despite the fact that it was a Saturday morning, Steve was able to contact Jerry at home. He told him about my crisis and Jerry dropped everything he was doing and made a house call.

He was able to restore calm. He convinced me to start taking an anti-depressant, and once again interceded in an almost impossible situation. This was not the last time I saw him as a therapist. Much more complicated situations would arise and Jerry would continue to assist me well beyond the turn of the Millennium, but those were still unanticipated issues.

Chapter 10

1996

Annus Horribilis

In 1992, Queen Elizabeth II, the monarch of the United Kingdom, described the year she had just had, her 40th as queen, as an annus horribilis, a Latin phrase meaning a horrible year. During that year a book was published chronicling the depression, dissatisfaction and disappointment of Diana, Princess of Wales, the wife of her son and heir, Charles, the Prince of Wales. There had been a disastrous fire in the Queen's favorite residence, Windsor Castle. And there was a growing disgruntled reaction of her subjects with her and her family.

Four years later I was facing my own annus horribilis. After a year of monthly travel, the chickens seemed to have come home to roost. I began 1996 with the desperate measures to try and stem the progress of the CMV retinitis that had been diagnosed in December of 1995. The IV ganciclovir infusions had not been effective. Unlike the IV pentamidine, where the treatments were once a day and the IV was removed immediately after the treatment, ganciclovir infusion was a twice daily infusion and one of the infusions had to be done at home when the Infusion Center was closed. But, my allergy to the latex in the needle necessary for the twice daily infusion tourniqueted and blocked this process. Therefore something other than infusion had to be found.

By January of 1996, Dr. Wolitz, my ophthalmologist was scrambling to find something that worked. His first solution was to give me intra-ocular injections, where he actually stabbed my eye with a syringe containing liquid ganciclovir. Unfortunately Cytomegalovirus (CMV) is an equal opportunity infection. In my case it had caused retinitis in my right eye. But it was just as likely to infect some other important organ so only injecting my eye could stop the retinitis there but it would leave the rest of my organs as great risk. This required an immediate solution so in lieu of infusions and injections, I was required to take 12 very large ganciclovir capsules.

But this was just one part of the mess. Because some friends who had moved to Honolulu had invited us to visit them in April we decided to take them up on their offer and go to Maui as well. Earlier in the year, our dog Wolfgang's epilepsy had taken a turn for the worse. He was experiencing many more fits and was starting to have difficulty getting to a place where he could have a bowel movement. Then he started to have difficulty walking and had to be assisted with a towel held under his belly in order to move anywhere. On March 28, 1996 my friend Walter drove me and Wolfgang to his veterinarian. We learned that in addition to his epilepsy Wolfgang was suffering from a rare form of cancer that was destroying his blood cells. The time had come for him to be euthanized.

The following date, March 29, 1996, Steve and I drove Wolfgang to his vet's office. I discovered that Steve and the vet had been conspiring behind my back to try and prolong Wolfgang's life as long as possible because they feared the reaction I would have to his loss. As devastating as I found his loss, I had been facing the loss of friends and my own impending death that I had to insist that I was totally opposed to extending any one's life, including Wolfgang's, for my own selfish reasons. Wolfgang's time was up and I refused to be an obstacle to that inevitable end.

In spite of the loss of Wolfgang we still took our planned trip to Hawaii. While we were in Hawaii we received a phone call from my former student, Valerie Leonard. Valerie called me to tell me that she would be making her Broadway debut in a secondary role in Oscar Wilde's *The Ideal Husband*. She expressed a hope and a desire that I come to see her in her debut, but qualified it saying that she would not be surprised if I wasn't able to fly to New York.

I was thrilled with the invitation and wondered if I might go, if I could afford the airfare, and find a place to stay. Several chapters ago I wrote about the suggested Thalidomide Study but I didn't mention the reason this had been suggested. The reason was that my Wasting Disease was progressing so fast that the problems with excessive diarrhea had increased exponentially and I was miserable. Some researchers felt that this abandoned drug which had been thought to be able to control the extreme nausea which accompanied pregnancy, might also be effective in controlling diarrhea in AIDS patients with wasting. I seemed to be the perfect candidate for this experiment.

So just before my May trip to New York to witness Valerie Leonard's Broadway debut I began taking Thalidomide.

I was deathly afraid of Thalidomide's side effects, but the diarrhea was getting so bad that I was at the point where I was willing to try anything. The principal Kaiser doctor doing the study was Dr. Fessel and he was very encouraging. Thalidomide did have an unfortunate side effect; it made me very sleepy which was somewhat dangerous for someone so ill who was planning on taking a cross-country flight by himself. Nevertheless I wanted to go to New York, I wanted to see Valerie's debut and I wanted to be free of diarrhea.

Everyone was wonderful to me during my trip to New York. Bruce Westcott, the brother of a close friend of mine, was an incredibly gracious host. In addition to getting me house seats for *An Ideal Husband*, Valerie treated me to a performance of *Rent*, the Broadway musical that adapted Puccini's *La Boheme*, giving it a rock beat and an AIDS message. *Rent* was incredibly difficult for me to watch, not only because it was telling my story, but because the Thalidomide was having no effect on my diarrhea and I spent most of the show running to the bathroom.

I returned from New York, grateful but exhausted. It did not take long for the Thalidomide Study folks to determine that the experiment had failed. It was not uncommon for my MHR AIDS Support volunteer Frank Blaikie to find me in tears when he came for our weekly visit because I had had so many diarrhea episodes before his arrival.

He tried to comfort me but my condition was making me very weak, very dehydrated, and very thin. I actually got down to 95 lbs. in contrast to my previous weight of 145 lbs. Losing 50 lbs. was a very big deal for a man with as small a frame as I have. Responding to my diminishing size and my problems with depression and excessive diarrhea, medically described as wasting, I was wasting away, Dr. Hill decided to try a tincture of opium regimen.

Unfortunately, just like the Thalidomide experiment, the tincture of opium trial did not do anything to stop my diarrhea. It did, however, exactly what one might expect from the tincture of opium. It generally anesthetized me to the point where I would fall asleep at the drop of a hat and respond to questions with very dopey answers. After all, tincture of opium is exactly that – dope.

I remember one afternoon when Steve and I visited my cousin Mark and his wife in the western part of Marin County. I was totally out of it during that visit, unresponsive, incoherent, or just asleep.

By the summer of 1996, many of my MHR AIDS Support Group brothers had started to take the most popular of the first protease inhibitor medications, Crixivan. After my many years of refusing to take any prophylactic AIDS medications, my doctor, my nurse practitioner, and Dr. Wolitz' nurse, Debra Thelen begged me to consider starting Crixivan. Reluctantly I did. But Crixivan had some really terrible side effects, principally, the very narrow window during which the medication could be taken was extremely restricting. If you didn't respect its idiosyncrasies, and sometimes it was impossible to do so, nausea and extreme projectile vomiting were the consequence. Any food eaten within two hours of taking Crixivan wrought havoc with one's digestive system. And if the food one ate had any fat, butter or oil, all bets were off. So in addition to wasting and terrible diarrhea I now had the devastating effects of Crixivan with no discernible benefit, all this was simply increasing my misery.

In the month of August, instead of making our usual vacation trip to the family Feather River Canyon vacation home, where we had had so much fun with our recently deceased dog Wolfgang, going to Graeagle involved too much pain, so we decided to choose a different destination. I hadn't been to the northern Sonoma Coast resort of Sea Ranch since childhood, and Steve had never been there. It seemed like a welcome opportunity to get away from San Francisco and have a relaxing time at a delightful resort.

But I was in no condition to enjoy a delightful resort. Once we arrived in our room at Sea Ranch I knew I had made a mistake. It's one thing to be sick and miserable at home. It's quite another to be in such a state in an unfamiliar place, to have to dress for meals in a restaurant and to be so uncomfortable that you would just as soon be dead.

But that is exactly what happened. I was unable to eat any meals, I spent more time on the toilet than anywhere else and I was absolutely unable to take walks on the beach with Steve or enjoy any of the simplest pleasures available at the resort.

Once we returned home after this weekend of misery I contacted Dr. Hill. He was well aware of how bad my situation was. My T-cells were still stuck at the zero level where they had been when the Thalidomide experiment began, just as they were when Dr. Hill started me on tincture of opium. It was clear that nothing was working. The protease inhibitor Crixivan was doing nothing to improve my condition and I was looking lasciviously at the knives in the kitchen as though they might be the solution to my misery. I had gotten to the point where I wanted out.

Dr. Hill, recognizing my despair, decided to take a different course. He decided that a strong course of morphine would be the solution. I was quite nervous about this decision and so he decided to hospitalize me so that any unfortunate consequences could be met with an immediate medical response.

The stay in the hospital began on September 12, 1996. In those days there were so many AIDS patients in San Francisco's Kaiser Facility that private rooms were out of the question. As I entered my room I had to pass by the bed of a very sick man, of course I too was a very sick man. By the following morning my roommate was dead. I have to say, they handled his death and removal very efficiently. I didn't even know that he had died or been removed, until I remarked on his empty bed and asked my nurse what had happened.

Dr. Hill had scheduled me for eight days in the hospital. I hate hospitals and it was very boring. I did have quite a few visitors however. A program called Godfathers, a group of Gay men who presented robes to patients with AIDS, brought me a robe. Since I was unable to attend my AIDS Support Group at our usual location, the men in my AIDS Support Group convened in my hospital room.

Steve and I have been attending the San Francisco Symphony concerts as subscribers for many years. The Symphony season begins in September, so our first concert fell during the weekend of my hospitalization. The first concert included one of my favorite pieces of classical music, Brahms Piano Concerto No. 1. I was so determined to attend this concert that I begged my doctor to give me permission to check out of the hospital, go home to shower and dress and then after attending the concert, sneak back into the hospital.

Well, I got my wish in spite of a total breach of usual hospital protocol, but the fact that I had so much morphine in my system meant I didn't hear much of the piano concerto. A doctor friend of mine was quite astonished that I had been able to pull off this caper, but the fact is my own doctor realized how important attendance at this concert was to me spiritually, despite the fact that I was asleep for most of the performance.

Before my hospitalization, Steve and I had planned a trip to Los Angeles to visit my brother and his family. Once I was back home from the hospital we realized that such an extensive automobile trip would not be the best thing for me given my very fragile condition. Instead we decided on a shorter trip to Monterey. We were able to find a very reasonable Bed and Breakfast in Pacific Grove, but when we got to Monterey, despite the fact that it was the first week in October, the daily temperatures were over 100^0. These high temperatures were hard on us and they were particularly hard on our Ford Escort's radiator. Add to that the soporific side effects of my heavy doses of morphine and you can imagine how this affected my enjoyment of our little vacation and by extension not to mention how it affected Steve's enjoyment. We returned home a little more miserable than the way we had left.

After the trip to Monterey I had several medical appointments, particularly one with my primary care giver, Dr. Hill and my ophthalmologist, Dr. Wolitz. I told them both that the morphine was doing little to stop my excessive diarrhea but it was having severe effects on my ability to breathe. During the course of many days I would find myself short of breath, unable to breathe. Dr. Hill suggested that I use a paper bag. I never was able to figure out the paper bag thing.

Steve was getting very uncomfortable leaving me at home alone as I was taking the morphine and having trouble breathing. He made a momentous decision, under President Clinton, the Family Medical Leave Act had been made law which allowed care givers like Steve to take time off from work and not lose their jobs.

One person who became particularly involved in my morphine problems was Dr. Wolitz' nurse Debra Thelen, the nurse who had encouraged me to try the Thalidomide Study and to start taking Crixivan. Learning of my problems with morphine she suggested that I see her friend Clarissa Ramstead. She told me that her friend Clarissa had some special techniques to assist those with breathing problems due to morphine. I welcomed any assistance with the morphine and breathing problems I was having. So we scheduled a meeting.

Debra and Clarissa came to see me at home several days later. The meeting began amicably enough with Clarissa asking me about my experiences since I had been diagnosed with AIDS. She asked me why Dr. Hill had prescribed morphine for me and why I had been hospitalized. She asked how I felt about these problems and what I wanted to do. I expressed my exhaustion and despair as I recounted my AIDS journey. Of course I told both of them about how I felt about the Crixivan and the fact that it was doing nothing for me aside from making me sicker.

I think by this point all of us were in tears. Clarissa began to comfort me and then explained what her job at Kaiser was. She told me that she was the principal nurse in Kaiser's Hospice Program. She said Hospice could alleviate many of my problems. My first reaction was: "Yeah Hospice will help me die," and I knew that despite my horrible condition, I was not yet ready *to die*, in spite of the fact that I had contemplated suicide many times over the past few months.

Clarissa's job and presentation scared me. She tried to convince me that Hospice would be a much more helpful program for me than that what was currently being done for me. She talked about organizing a group of my friends and relatives to assist Steve in Caring for me. She told me that despite the fact that Hospice was a program of palliative care to assist those for whom ordinary medicine was no longer an effective means of keeping a patient alive it might work for me. She told me that it was designed to provide a dignified death to those for whom there were no solutions. Nevertheless, because of the experimental nature of protease inhibitors I would be allowed to continue taking them. I would also be allowed to continue my treatments for CMV retinitis and the other opportunistic infections which were plaguing me.

My reaction at first was: "Yeah, it sounds great but I don't want to die and going into Hospice means I have to accept I am dying." Her response was, "Why don't you try it and see if it works for you, if it doesn't you can always quit."

Reluctantly, I consented. I felt like I had been "Shanghaied" by these kind ladies. But at that point I really had no other options. Once I gave them my reluctant assent the details were presented. Clarissa told me that in addition to the extra care I would receive by entering Hospice care, Steve would also benefit. Clarissa would arrange a special meeting with the friends and relatives I thought would be willing to help me in what appeared to be my final transition. She told me that the actual entrance into Hospice would be accomplished in a meeting between me and my doctor, where many documents would be signed and filed. She told me that two special benefits to me in addition to her weekly home visits would be three visits a week from a home-health aide who would assist me with personal care and massage, and a Hospice Volunteer who would provide emotional support on a weekly basis. The special care I would be getting sounded great. Even though I already had volunteer support from a Shanti Volunteer and a Most Holy Redeemer's AIDS Support Group Volunteer, I also very much looked forward to having the Hospice Emotional Support Volunteer.

After the ten months of the Annus Horribilis of 1996, in spite of the fact that I was entering a palliative care program to help me prepare for death, it felt like things were looking up at last.

Chapter 11

Hospice

With my meeting with Clarissa finished, I knew what the next steps would be. First there was the post Hospice interview meeting with my doctor. He confessed that he thought it was time for me to enter Hospice care but he had been reluctant to broach the subject, expressing gratitude for Debra and Clarissa's intervention. Dr. Hill, in addition to all the other members of my health care team, was quite aware of the ineffectiveness of the protease inhibitors in ameliorating my AIDS conditions. The point at which the "Hospice" suggestion is made to a patient is probably one of the most difficult moments in a doctor's relationship with his patient. During the appointment with Dr. Hill it was made quite clear that my Hospice experience would be very different from someone who had something like inoperable cancer. I would continue to see all my regular specialists along with Dr. Hill himself. My drug regimen would not change, even the protease inhibitors would continue.

The second thing that happened was that I gave Clarissa a list of my friends and relatives who had indicated to me that they would be willing to be an integral part of my care team; that they would be available to stay with me when Steve needed to do an errand or take a break. The gathering happened shortly after my appointment with Dr. Hill and Clarissa's receipt of my potential caregiver list. There were at least twenty friends and relatives who attended this meeting. Clarissa told them that I was entering a period of transition which would probably end with my death. It was a sobering moment for me, Steve, my friends and relatives. But everyone was willing to face this reality with me. The meeting ended with hugs, eyes near tears and very comforting words, but we were off and running.

My weekly visits with Clarissa began immediately. She came to our house shortly after breakfast and tested all my vital signs, took many vials of blood, and gave me an overall assessment of my health condition. At the first meeting she introduced me to my Home Health Aide, William. William also worked as a patient aide at UCSF. He was a very kind and caring man with a warm sense of humor. He gave me a bath, trimmed my hair and nails and gave me a massage. I felt much better after he left. I looked forward to his thrice weekly visits. I was beginning to think that being a Hospice patient was not so bad.

The next thing that happened with regard to Hospice was my introduction to my Hospice Emotional Support Volunteer, Dennis Setlock. Dennis worked for the Federal Government. He was able to get time off from work every week for our emotional support visits. Dennis had lost the man, with whom he had a long-term relationship, to AIDS several years before he decided to do volunteer work. The first question I asked Dennis was would he be willing to help me with my share of the housekeeping. Dennis had no difficulty in telling me that he was not available for such chores but he was more than willing to take me on various out of home excursions. He liked movies and I like movies so we decided to start by going to movies in his 1960's red

Mustang convertible. Over the years we were together, Dennis and I went to movies, medical appointments, and when my health improved, swimming outings.

My Hospice journey began benignly enough. There were many things I liked. The medical and personal care were incredible. My relationship with Dennis flowered and we always had fun when we went to the movies. Gradually, as November 1996 slid into December and the month of Christmas, my health problems were still getting worse but that of course was expected for patients under Hospice care. As my immune system deteriorated my skin and scalp problems proceeded to get worse and worse. Dr. Goldstein had no effective solutions and Clarissa was trying anything she thought might work. At one point we all quoted the *Star Wars* line, "Help me Obi-Wan Kenobi, you're my only hope." Things had actually gotten that bad, but again, I *was* a Hospice patient.

In spite of the great Hospice care I was receiving and the protease inhibitors I was taking things kept getting worse and I was trying to put the best face on it. In December Steve and I still held our Christmas party with carols and lots of desserts. We joined my family in Santa Rosa for prime rib and gifts on Christmas Day. On December 28, 1996 we remembered celebrating our 10th Anniversary with a big party the year before, but it looked pretty bleak and I was.

I was still dealing with emotional issues with my therapist, Jerry Geffner. I was seeing him about once a month at this point and my December appointment came a few weeks before Christmas. I guess I looked like I was at death's door and Jerry looked startled when he saw me. He particularly wanted me to know that he was going to Central America for an extended stay. He didn't say goodbye as though he wouldn't see me again, but years later he confessed to me that that's what he was thinking.

When 1997 began I started to take a turn for the worse. I suppose it was partially a combination of depression, morphine and falling T-cells. As all these hopeless moments were concatenating, the consequence of spending Christmas in the presence of my young nieces and nephews was that I was diagnosed with pneumonia, not pneumocystis pneumonia but just the ordinary pneumonia of the elderly and idle. My mother always called it the "old peoples' friend." It was marked by lung congestion, lots of coughing and overall malaise. During most of January I was confined to my bed. One of my friends actually was willing to read from a novel which was the current selection of my Trollope Reading Group.

January 1997 had the distinction of combining President Clinton's "State of the Union Speech" with the split screen coverage of the verdict in the O.J. Simpson Civil Trial. My cousin, Mark Brown, one of the group of volunteers which had been assembled by Clarissa, joined me on that incredible television night.

As January progressed, my condition was worsening and I could see no light at the end of the tunnel. I began to ask myself why I was putting myself through this torture. During the pneumonia infection I asked my astrologer friend, Jack Fertig, if he would come to my house and do a reading. The night he came I was so sick and the weather was so stormy that the power went out during Jack's reading. He told me that my prognosis was bleak. It was hardly news to me. He told me I would have to pass through the astrological equivalent of the "eye of a needle." I wasn't rich and I am not a camel but I had heard that Biblical expression before.

In the days after this reading, as January passed into February, I talked to a friend Walter, from my MHR AIDS Support Group. We had watched many friends from our group die and I told him I thought I was ready to join them. I told him I didn't think I could tolerate any more drugs and that they just were not working. As our conversation continued while standing in the garden enjoying my plants and the early February sun, it became clear that what I was doing was not making any sense. Gradually, as it developed in my mind I told Walter I was going to stop all medications and let my disease take over. I was very sad but very determined.

That night, the first Thursday in February 1997, I decided I had to tell Steve. He had watched me deteriorate during my first three years with AIDS. He had supported me through all the crises and he knew how exhausting the last year had been for me. It had been just as frustrating and exhausting for him.

After we had eaten dinner, I summoned the courage to tell Steve that I had made a decision to stop taking all medications. I was so tired of their side effects and the fact that they were doing nothing to change my failing condition. The dreadful experience of the past month's pneumonia had sealed the deal. I was sick of being sick and I just didn't think I could keep fighting with no sense of improved health. I could see how crushed he was by my statement.

We decided to watch what we thought would be a completely innocuous program. It was a special program about the Broadway and Pop singer, Elaine Paige, the British actress was featured in *Sunset Boulevard, Cats! Chess,* and a one woman show about the French chanteuse Edith Piaf. The light hearted nature of the show eased our depressed mood and we were both enjoying the show until it got to the last section, the Edith Piaf set. The Piaf song set recalled the feelings we both had experienced while discussing the termination of all medications and by implication my life. Finally, the song lyric, "If you love me, whatever happens I don't care," brought an uncontrollable flow of tears. We knew that the next day would bring Clarissa and that it would be a prime opportunity to bring this problem to a conclusion.

We went to bed very sad. We had struggled with my complicated AIDS condition trying to put a good face on a frequently hopeless situation. Meeting Clarissa for my regular appointment loomed in our minds before her arrival. When Clarissa arrived we greeted her with our most ebullient faces. We had our usual vital sign tests, blood draws, and an overall assessment of my current health. Then I dropped the bomb. As hard as it was to tell her, I said that after the horrible month of January and the pneumonia accompanying it I had come to the conclusion that the battle was over that I was ready to stop all medications and just prepare myself to die.

Surprisingly, despite the fact that Clarissa was the one who had convinced me to enter Hospice, her first statement was, "Frank, give me one more week." I wondered, since nothing positive had happened so far, what could possibly change in a week? At that point I begrudgingly decided to give her that week.

Befuddled, I wondered what the week would bring me. Perhaps Clarissa had seen some other patients begin to show improvements as the protease inhibitors affected them. As Clarissa and I were waiting for the following Friday, Steve found an enzyme in a health food store in the Castro and suggested that I start taking it.

Amazingly, whether it was the enzyme from the health food store or the protease inhibitor finally providing me with relief or just my body advancing after the most recent bout of pneumonia, something changed. By the time Clarissa visited me on the second Friday of February I had lost my desire to "go off all medications," I had decided to give Clarissa more than the week she had asked. On the other hand I must state that I was still in very bad shape.

There was no way I was going to be released from Hospice. My T-cells could still be counted on one hand if that. And my viral load, indicating the amount of virus still attacking my body and immune system, was still astronomical.

In the meanwhile, in spite of the fact that I was a Hospice patient I was still regularly seeing Dr. Wolitz, my ophthalmologist, and Dr. Goldstein, my dermatologist. When my therapist, Jerry Geffner, returned from Central America, he was very relieved to hear that I was still alive, but regrettably he had to inform me that he was changing jobs and could no longer serve as my therapist. We were both very sad about this development.

I was still extremely fragile, my relationship with my Hospice volunteer, Dennis, (we had developed a pattern of going to movies that were having their first screenings on Friday) was going great. As I began to regain strength, Dennis and I returned to the YMCA to test whether I still had the strength to swim. It was the first time I had been able to swim since before my hospitalization in September 1996.

My birthday is in February, and although 45 is not a particularly important birthday, Steve planned a surprise birthday party in gratitude that I had had such a dramatic turnaround. I was definitely very weak, but heartened by the love and support I received from my friends and some of my family. It was definitely an unexpected birthday by me and by all the guests, but it happened and it actually looked like I had turned a corner.

At this point my health care team was cautiously optimistic, after all I had been hospitalized just five months before the birthday and had started taking morphine, usually a drug used by hospice teams to ease the pains associated with dying. In November my condition was so severe that I was tricked into Hospice. In January my condition had weakened to the point where I succumbed to ordinary pneumonia. At the beginning of February I had reached a point of despair so severe that I had decided to stop all medications and let nature take its course. But with my birthday in my rear view mirror, I decided to start taking some risks.

The extreme weakness that had resulted from my AIDS conditions and from my time in Hospice made going to the "Y" a risk, but the results were amazing. Just going to the Y and attempting to swim were worth all the exhaustion I had endured. But, in one more way I had turned a corner.

As a consequence of all this progress, you might think these would have been powerful reasons for ending my time in Hospice, my death sentence. They were neither; Dr. Hill, Clarissa and my T-cells had indicated and seen enough recovery to allow me to be released from Hospice.

The various protease inhibitors, and they were many, in sequential single dose fashion, had some very curious results occurring with them. A very gradual increase of T-cells was happening only to be followed by a crash. They would go up then just as quickly go down. And they were not having any effect on my many AIDS related opportunistic infections.

In spite of going into Hospice, my regular visits to Dr. Wolitz for my on-going CMV Retinitis continued. I had consented to be part of a study to investigate the effectiveness of an experimental treatment for the retinitis. It was not doing anything for the CMV Retinitis, but it did involve weekly visits, examinations and very painful photographs of my dilated eyes and retina.

Then something really unexpected happened. I began to experience the same symptoms I had had in 1994 when I was diagnosed with diabetes. Since somehow my exercise regime before I was placed into Hospice I had actually corrected my diabetes, I thought it was over. I reported these diabetes symptoms to my doctor and the tests he made confirmed that once again I had diabetes. I asked Dr. Hill if the symptoms could be caused by whichever protease inhibitor I was taking. He almost categorically refuted my suspicions. The very next day in *The San Francisco Chronicle* I read an article saying that researchers in New England had discovered the relationship between protease inhibitors and the presence of diabetes.

I brought this information to Dr. Hill and he reacted with skeptical raised eyebrows, nevertheless, he sent me for a blood test and the blood test confirmed that the diabetes, which I thought had been conquered, was back. I immediately was put back on twice daily insulin and rejoined the very rocky road of diabetes care management.

But I was still an AIDS patient whose condition was so severe that he had been placed in hospice care. It almost became something worthy of an asterisk, as in "Oh, yeah, in addition to all his life threatening diseases, Frank also has diabetes, but we've got much bigger fish to fry." My diabetes was an additional annoyance, but not problem number one. I would be referred to Diabetic Educators, but I didn't take diabetes or them very seriously. I was still very angry about having diabetes and very uncooperative in regard to my own diabetic care.

As 1997 progressed so did I in my recovery. Although it probably was time for me to exit hospice care, I didn't want to. I liked the extra attention, the free drugs, and the other perks, like William's special personal care, my Hospice AIDS Volunteer, Dennis, and the free taxi vouchers which made it easier for me to get around the city. After my visit to the YMCA for a swim with Dennis, I gradually resumed my swimming. I even started riding my bike to the "Y."

Then on the day Diana, Princess of Wales, was killed in a car crash in Paris, something awful happened to me. On that Sunday afternoon, August 31, 1997, I was riding my bike to the "Y" and turned left off of Market Street onto Laguna. Though most streets in San Francisco are crowned for drainage, the intersection I was crossing was crowned higher than most. I came off the curb, riding in the crosswalk, too quickly. The bounce of the bike and my body caused my sternum to be thrown into the nut in the middle of the bike's handlebar. The pain was extraordinary, but instead of stopping and dealing with the pain, I chose to bike the several miles still necessary to reach the "Y." I thought I would still be able to swim. I was wrong. I had to call Steve and ask him to pick me and my bike up. When he arrived he realized what incredible pain I was experiencing.

Steve drove me and my bike to Kaiser San Francisco's Emergency Room. Sunday afternoon is a pretty quiet time at that Emergency Room and I was seen, triaged and x-rayed very quickly. The emergency room doctor confirmed that I had sustained a hairline fracture in my sternum. I suppose hairline fractures in other body parts hurt, but in the sternum the pain is extraordinary. I was told that there was nothing that could be done to promote healing other than rest, rest, rest. Breathing hurt, coughing hurt, any movement hurt. I could not lie prone to sleep but had to sit up in bed. This accident was followed by a very slow recovery.

By October I was healed enough to return to the "Y" to swim. I was leery about getting back on my bike. I was still practicing the yoyo game with protease inhibitors and my T-cells, up and down and each time I would be changed to a new protease inhibitor. But in 1997 Dr. Hill and I were running out of options. First of all there were a lot fewer protease inhibitors than there are nineteen years later.

Also once the virus mutated to become resistant to the inhibitor that inhibitor could no longer be used. Despite the fact that my health had been improving from the point I had entered Hospice, everyone determined that the fragility of my condition warranted my remaining under hospice care.

Around this point, my wonderful hospice nurse, Clarissa, had decided to return to UCSF to get her Nurse Practitioner degree and license. My new case manager was not as friendly or supportive as Clarissa had been and she really wanted me out of Hospice. In 2012 I discovered while my mother was under hospice care that Medicare and everyone else expects a hospice patient to be dead after six months of care. By six months I was not only still alive but a lot better than I had been. By November they really wanted me dead or out of Hospice. I dragged my feet as much as possible. I even had a bad case of erysipelas, a life threatening blood disorder. I felt that staying on hospice was still appropriate.

Then something totally unexpected happened. My very compassionate and unique (at one point, the only San Francisco Kaiser doctor who was willing to treat AIDS patients doctor, Dr. Hill had had enough; enough bureaucratic red tape, enough patients dying under his care, enough of Kaiser. As I reached my year anniversary in Hospice he decided to retire.

Changing primary care providers is a very traumatic event. Making the change while being under hospice care, wondering from one moment to the next when "the next shoe will drop" is terrifying. By this point another doctor had become an active researcher and provider for AIDS patients. His name was Dr. Fessel and he was the doctor and primary researcher on the Thalidomide study in which I had participated. Dr. Hill thought he might be a good fit for me. I started to see him and one of the strangest things he did was to attempt to treat my problem with diabetes with a higher dose of insulin which made me so hungry that I was having to eat five bowls of cereal at breakfast just to start the day.

Because of the effect of pentamidine on my pancreas during my three IV treatments for pneumocystis, I was having a very difficult time absorbing fat, I had had wasting syndrome and was very thin. Because of this, one of my health care providers suggested that I join a study at UCSF's San Francisco General Hospital which tested whether using an insulin pump which time released measured doses of pancreatic enzymes would help me with the wasting. The primitive insulin pump and the pancreatic enzyme did not work, but like anything else in the hit or miss world of AIDS research it seemed to be worth a try. The fact that the insulin pump was so painful would eventually have a deleterious effect on me in the years to come.

During the time that I was seeing Dr. Fessel another new doctor joined the Kaiser AIDS health care team. His arrival had been inspired by his new acquaintance with my ophthalmologist, Dr. Wolitz. Dr. Stephen Follansbee had been in private practice and a prominent research scientist advancing solutions for AIDS patients. He had become exhausted by the non-medical costs of medical care. Dr. Wolitz had recommended him to the Kaiser Board and he was welcomed just at the point that Dr. Hill retired. For the first several months after Hill's retirement I was seen by both.

Simultaneously, a new approach to the care of AIDS patients had been revealed as being incredibly successful with patients in Germany. The game changing idea was to attack the AIDS retrovirus with a multi-drug therapy instead of one at time until the drug failed in a single drug therapy.

By February I had chosen Dr. Follansbee as my primary care physician and he had started me on my first AIDS drug "cocktail." The term cocktail was used because it was a mix of four drugs. Each was supposed to attack the retro-virus at different stages of the viral life, cell division, recombination, integration and so on.

Because I was at risk for failure of this combination therapy, I still insisted that I remain a hospice patient. The Kaiser Hospice team was not happy about this request but Dr. Follansbee supported me. I remained a Hospice patient in early 1998.

I was very happy about the changes that were happening in my life and health. I still had my cab vouchers which meant I could still travel by cab for free. On Saturday, February 14, 1998, I decided to cab to the YMCA to go swimming in the afternoon, and then go to the hotel which I knew had a cab-stand in its garage. I should have known that Valentine's Day on a Saturday would be a dreadful afternoon to get a cab. It was. I waited a full hour and got hotter and hotter as I kept calling the cab company asking for a cab. Finally, a cab came.

It is a well-known fact that hotel cab stands are frequented by cab drivers who want to take passengers to the airport for a very healthy fare. In addition cab drivers hate cab vouchers. And the streets were filled Valentine's revelers and these streets were hard to negotiate.

When my cab driver arrived I was already as annoyed as he was. Instead of keeping my mouth shut and being grateful that he arrived to drive me home, I started complaining about the hour I had waited; he became more annoyed. He was annoyed about the fact that I was giving him a lousy voucher fare and that he would be mired in city traffic. He also seemed to be annoyed by the fact that I was not Asian like him, and at least presented as being Gay.

Instead of just doing his job and driving me home he called me a "faggot" and ratcheted up an already tense situation. I responded pejoratively to his tremendously inflammatory label. Suddenly, instead of continuing down Gough Street to Market to drive me home, he made an erratic turn onto Grove Street stopped the cab very quickly, rushed around to the passenger back door, pulled me out of his cab, and violently threw me against the curb. The shock and the pain were unbearable. As I writhed on the sidewalk he sped away. After receiving some assistance from a passerby I was able to get to my feet and use my cell phone to call Steve. While I nursed my wounds he tried to get me to the Kaiser Emergency Room as quickly as possible, again having to navigate the heavy Valentine Saturday night traffic.

Once Steve picked me up, he took me to Kaiser's Emergency Room. I was quickly triaged and sent for x-rays. Despite my pain, the x-rays showed no broken bones and tissue bruising is hard to identify and record until several days have passed and the bruises are revealed.

I was sent home angry, disappointed, and wanted revenge. I made a report to the Castro's CUAV, the Community United Against Violence. CUAV suggested that I contact a lawyer and pursue my quest for justice, or should I say revenge.

I had no idea which lawyer I would choose. My friends at the Most Holy Redeemer AIDS Support Group suggested I seek counsel from an attorney who had a one man practice on Noe Street. I made an appointment and he felt I had a case. He was particularly interested in using the Gay Anti-Discrimination Hate Crime Law. If that law worked in my favor the financial judgment would be tripled. Both of our sets of eyes bulged with greed.

I was pretty naïve about how law suits and courts work, about how long something like this would last, about how much painful stress it would cause, about being put under hostile cross examination, and about alienating a jury.

By the time the case went to trial I had long ago graduated from Hospice, but I include it in the Hospice chapter because it began while I was still in Hospice and still using my Hospice cab vouchers.

Once we went to trial I should have seen the handwriting on the wall. Before we even chose a jury, the cab company tried to settle for a generous sum of $10,000. The judge practically begged me to take the deal. My attorney, however, still had eyes the size of saucers and they were filled with dollar signs tripled because of the hate crime law. Against my better judgment but still driven by greed and revenge I decided to take the plunge. Despite the fact that Jerry Geffner was no longer my Kaiser therapist, my lawyer used him as a character witness for me trying to garner sympathy.

Everything backfired, my lawyer's friend told him before his final argument that he was going to lose the case. The attorney for the cab company who had taken my deposition disappeared once the jury was selected. He was replaced by a Chinese lawyer defending the Chinese cab driver, and had no problem attacking me and making me the cause of the argument that precipitated my injury, something unlikely to have been done by the Caucasian suburban and possibly Gay lawyer who had taken my deposition.

The Ace won, we lost. Since my lawyer had taken my case without any kind of retainer expecting a big 40% fee from my settlement his loss had to be paid for by someone and that someone was yours truly. It just added insult to injury and I had learned a very painful lesson.

But there were a lot of other things that happened in 1998 besides the accident. Even though I was showing many signs of improvement, I was very concerned about what might happen as I started the new four drug combination which for me was otherwise known as the "AIDS cocktail," and might have some unexpected side-effects. After all I had become famous in Kaiser AIDS care circles for being allergic to almost every other drug I took. I used this factor to sustain my claim to still be eligible for Hospice care. It worked; the powers that be rolled their eyes but allowed me to stay. By this point I had chosen Dr. Follansbee as my primary care physician and he supported my claim to still need Kaiser's Hospice care. I think he assumed that a couple of months on the "cocktail" would turn the tide and my eligibility for Hospice would become moot. I think he thought that two more months of Hospice would be preferable to a battle.

Even though Clarissa had left Kaiser Hospice to get her Nurse Practitioner degree at UCSF, she agreed to participate in my official end of Hospice care. Steve and I organized a special graduation party. We invited all those who had participated in my care as Hospice Caregivers, plus my parents, family and friends. I had never attended a party like this one let alone been feted at one. Aside from hors d'oeuvres, a cake, a beautiful weather day, and pleasant conversation, the pinnacle of the party's festivities was the moment when Clarissa and I decked out with angels' wings came center stage and Clarissa demanded that I return my wings. There were cheers, tears, smiles, laughter and hugs. We were all so happy and shocked that this day had arrived. My presumed death had been postponed.

Fourteen months prior to this celebration when I had decided to stop taking any medication, Steve had told me that if I got better he would take me to Europe or at least Italy. As I had graduated from Hospice, something I had hardly expected when he made the promise, we planned our Italian trip.

Like our other trips to Europe we would travel for three weeks. We flew to Milan, picked up our rental car, drove to Verona, then Venice. Next was Rossini's hometown of Pesaro. From Pesaro we drove across the Gran Sasso d'Italia to L'Aquila then visited the ancient Benedictine Monastery of Monte Cassino. From central Italy we proceeded to the Salerno area where my Italian cousins lived. After visits to Sorrento, Capri and Amalfi we returned to the north and stopped in Florence. I had to pay a return visit to the step where I had broken down in tears in 1993 thinking that I would never see Florence again. Our trip was almost over and then we returned to Milan for our return flight.

The Italian trip had been a fitting celebration marking my graduation from Hospice. At this point I had to face a new reality. I was no longer dying, at least quickly enough to be a Hospice patient. What I was experiencing now had a name, "the Lazarus Effect." I don't know what kind of life Lazarus lived after Jesus called him back from death. But in a way my journey reminds me more of Dr. Manette's release from the Bastille in Charles Dickens *A Tale of Two Cities*, than the Lazarus experience. I now had to recreate my life. That's the rest of this story.

Chapter 12

After Hospice

My graduation from Hospice happened on a beautiful Sunday in May. I had friends, family, medical workers, and those who had helped Steve bring me through my Hospice journey. But after the graduation and the trip to Italy I had to start living my life. I still had many of the problems I had had before I entered Hospice. I still saw my dermatologist regularly. I still saw my ophthalmologist; my vision was still at risk. Before I had entered Hospice my medical team had decided that it was no longer safe for me to be infused with pentamidine when I had one of my many episodes of pneumocystis pneumonia, and there were several more. Despite the fact that I had an allergic reaction to Septra, the most effective oral drug to prevent pneumocystis, there was a protocol for patients like me. It was called Septra desensitization. By titrating very minimal amounts of the drug gradually over several weeks, doubling the dose progressively, the process made it possible for me to take the drug without the allergic reaction. Everyone hoped that this would stop the pneumocystis flare-ups. The "AIDS cocktail" did end the problems with CMV infection and ended my weekly appointments with my ophthalmologist.

I still had many appointments with my Dermatologist. As my health improved I really began to think I might even return to the work force. Because my job as a Consulting Systems Engineer, a fancy Bank of America name for a computer programmer, the five years that had elapsed since I went on permanent disability was exponentially longer than the five calendar years in the systems engineering world. I was so behind the curve that it was unlikely that I would ever be able to catch up. I decided to make a complete career change. Despite the fact that the Bay Area is glutted with psychologists and psychotherapists, I decided that I would try this anyway.

In the summer of 1998, four months after my graduation from Hospice, I decided that it was time for me to go back to school. Jerry Geffner was no longer in a position to counsel me. The person who did counsel me advised me to think seriously about making this move. She told me that I might possibly lose my entire Kaiser and other benefits. But I was determined. I registered at San Francisco State as an undergraduate. I registered with the AIDS foundation to take a training course to become a counselor to reveal results of HIV tests. I hoped that this would firm up my bona fides to become a psychotherapist.

I started the course at the AIDS Foundation in August. I started SF State in September. By October the rigors of class and training had taken their toll. I once again succumbed to pneumocystis in spite of the Septra prophylaxis. Since Dr. Follansbee was on vacation, I was treated by Dr. Gold. She prescribed rest and increased my Septra dose and vigorously encouraged me to forget about re-enrolling in college. This temporary plan was shelved with little hope of return.

And I was once again at sea as to what to do with my life. Once I recovered from my fifth pneumocystis bout I continued to do what I had been doing before deciding to investigate returning to college. I structured my days around a regular workout schedule using the stationary bike at the YMCA. During my more fragile days before I entered Hospice I had made a resolution with myself that no matter how bad I felt in the morning I would force myself to get out of the house saying that I might look back on the so-called "bad day" and wished I had felt as good as I felt on that "bad" day. This allowed me to do things which I might not have done otherwise.

I continued to enjoy the company of my three support volunteers, the person from Shanti, my Most Holy Redeemer AIDS Support Group volunteer, and despite the fact that I was no longer a Kaiser Hospice patient, my relationship with my Kaiser Hospice volunteer, he and I continued to go to movies on Fridays unless I had an appointment to which he would take me. These volunteers punctuated my week, but when I had no appointment or volunteer I went to the "Y" and enjoyed my books and CDs and records. In the evening I enjoyed my vast video collection.

I imagine that regimen sounds pretty boring but that is what I was doing. My medical appointments lessened after the AIDS "cocktail" started working. Then in January 1999 something very unexpected happened. Since the "cocktail" seemed to be working, stopping my almost weekly visits to my ophthalmologist and dermatologist, I no longer needed to take medication to prevent CMV retinitis, my own higher T-cells were protecting me as they should. The thing that happened that was surprising was that I began to have neurological problems. I had terrific problems with balance. I was frequently falling down. I was having trouble finding words while I was speaking. And when I was writing I would drop the second letter whenever a double letter occurred in a word.

These sudden neurological changes were very frightening. I reported them to Dr. Follansbee at my next appointment and we speculated that I might have developed a case of PML, Progressive Multi-focal Leukoencephalopathy. PML is undoubtedly the very worst of the opportunistic infections made possible by the AIDS virus. Among other things it would be necessary for one's T-cells to be very very low for even the possibility of infection with PML to take place. After taking the AIDS "cocktail" for over a year it was particularly surprising for me to even be considered as a person with PML.

The really bad news about PML was that the life expectancy after diagnosis was no more than six weeks. Steve and I were terrified. I had survived many opportunistic infections and a stint in Hospice, so with the possibility of PML and my immediate demise we were sent into a tremendous depression.

With all this in mind Dr. Follansbee had sent me to a neurologist. The neurologist ordered an MRI of my brain and when we reviewed the findings the immediate presumptive diagnosis was PML, but absolute confirmation would require a sampling of the fluid in my brain. The places where the lesions showed in my brain were the areas governing speech, balance, and interaction of vocabulary and spelling, exactly what I had been experiencing.

As I was contemplating my resistance to having the brain fluid tested, Dr. Follansbee came to my rescue. Since he was not only a doctor but an AIDS research scientist it is not surprising that he was aware that brain and mental problems had been occurring in AIDS patients taking Sustiva, as one of the drugs in their "cocktails." He suggested that instead of drawing the brain or spinal fluid that I simply stop taking Sustiva. After two weeks off the drug my brain showed improvement. Steve and I were so grateful that I didn't have PML. Dr. Follansbee still had to find a drug to replace the evil Sustiva but that didn't seem as difficult as dealing with a disease that was guaranteed to kill me in six weeks.

I had dodged another bullet, but there were many more waiting for me. Particularly daunting was my difficulty in controlling my blood sugars and dealing with the increasing challenges caused by skin cancers. Additionally I was continuing to have chronic diarrhea.

Chapter 13

Out of Control

Diabetes

My diabetes diagnosis was due to the fact that two successive treatments with pentamidine had destroyed my pancreas. In 1993 there was no better alternative for me than pentamidine to treat the pneumocystis pneumonia that was threatening my life. I had had many friends who had succumbed to this disease and despite the extreme rigors of this IV drug; I had been treated with it twice. The second treatment led to kidney problems and eventually the destruction of my pancreas. The pancreas among other things holds the very important islets of Langerhans, the organs that manufacture insulin (Insula is the Latin word for islands. Islets is an English word meaning small island hence the Islets of Langerhans are an archipelago near the pancreas where insulin is produced). Insulin is the vital substance that allows sugar to nourish the cells. Without insulin the cell doors remain locked so that sugar cannot nourish the cells and instead simply is excreted in urine. The results are terrible; the kidneys become overtaxed, weight loss is almost guaranteed and eventually the resulting anemia leads to both weakness and poor production of red blood cells, hence anemia.

When I was diagnosed with diabetes, following the failure of my pancreas, the subsequent weight loss and higher levels of blood sugar upset me very much. I thought, isn't AIDS enough, do I really need diabetes too? I was also furious because eleven years prior, in an attempt to improve my health, I had completely eliminated sugar from my diet. The diabetes seemed grossly unfair.

Partially because of my sense of the unfairness of the diagnosis I became the least cooperative diabetic patient ever. Driven by anger I started to make up for my abstinence from sugar by eating as much sugar as I could. I completely changed my approach to sugar. I had candy, sugared sodas, and desserts whenever possible. I felt that since my principle diagnosis was AIDS, diabetes was just an "and" disease, and that I would probably die before any serious consequences of diabetes; ridiculous sugar binging resulted.

I did occasionally try to adhere to the guidelines presented to me by my healthcare professionals, but usually I was resentful, angry and uncooperative. Many of these professionals would ask me to keep track of what I ate and I pretended to follow their directions. I made bogus reports of the very balanced sugar free meals I had eaten. Every time I met with these professionals I felt like I had been summoned to the Dean's office for a reprimand. These meetings were horrible for me and probably for the professionals as well. Since blood tests never lie, and the professionals had the test results before them, they knew that I was lying – to them and to myself.

There is a test, beyond the simple blood glucose test, called the hemoglobin A1C test. This test somehow is able to provide a snapshot of the average of one's blood sugars over the past three months. A good number showing effective blood sugar control is 6.0, mine was in the range of 10.0 to 12.0 – very bad and dangerous. And in spite of these numbers I continued to lie and attempt to eat sugar to my own destruction.

Among the abetting factors were the unexpected effects of the protease inhibitors on blood sugar and on cholesterol. So the combination of a failed pancreas, protease inhibitors, and my anger and reluctance to be a cooperative diabetic patient was a recipe for disaster.

One of the more disconcerting effects of poor diabetic management is the dangerous and sometimes deadly condition called hypoglycemia. Hypoglycemia happens when blood sugar falls so low, many debilitating things occur. As blood sugar falls the first thing manifested is irritability, sometimes to the point of combativeness. This is usually followed by confusion and disorientation. And finally the worst effect is loss of consciousness and at the same time loss of blood cells. Sometimes these hypoglycemic events can also be complicated with seizures which can be accompanied with bone fractures and concussions.

There is also the polar opposite of diabetic problems – hyperglycemia. When one's blood sugar is astronomically high instead of abysmally low, hyperglycemia happens. That too can lead to a coma or the deadly ketoacidosis. These two conditions, which usually precede and follow each other, result in another unfortunate condition known as hypoglycemia unawareness. For those who have an ordinary functioning endocrine system which automatically informs one's consciousness that he is having a low blood sugar, i.e., hypoglycemia, the results are a ravenous appetite which demands food, carbohydrates and sugar to correct this dangerous condition. However, when a brittle diabetic experiences the swings from uncontrolled blood sugar that lead to hypoglycemia and hyperglycemia, the so-called hypoglycemia awareness gradually recedes until the diabetic has no hypoglycemic awareness at all.

All this technical stuff is background to what was happening to me. I've told you how unhappy I was about my diagnosis of diabetes. I have told you how uncooperative I was with my diabetic caregivers and how I continually lied about the causes of my skyrocketing Hemoglobin A1c readings. They knew I was lying and I knew I was lying but nobody wanted to identify the liar or the lies. So we just continued to limp along but I was experiencing more and more hypoglycemic unawareness, more and more lows that resulted in dizziness, unpleasant all over body sweating, and loss of consciousness, plus many rescues by 911 first responders who ultimately would take me by ambulance to the emergency room.

I had ceased to be an AIDS patient who happened to have brittle diabetes and became a brittle diabetic who happened to have an AIDS diagnosis. The actual solutions to these frightening issues will be discussed in a later chapter concomitant with other issues. For the moment it should be understood that my diabetic issues were exacerbated by excessive consumption of sugared beverages. This happened most frequently when we visited our friends in the Sierra foothills. While staying at their house for several days and excessively consuming these sugared sodas, at night I had to get up practically every hour in order to urinate. I hated it, but I was unwilling to do the necessary footwork to address this issue. I was unwilling to stop drinking my beloved overly sweet sugared sodas, my anger and lack of cooperation about diabetes was feeding my intransigence and I didn't think there would be any other consequences.

Chapter 14

Dr. Goldstein

And Skin Cancer

When I was a child, (I was born in 1952), there was little or no concern about the dangerous ultra-violet rays that accompanied sun exposure. Naturally, parents protected infants from too much sun exposure, but even as a little baby in a stroller my mother would frequently push me without sun protection and when we'd vacation in Healdsburg on the Russian River suntan lotion usually was applied but never sun screen. From childhood to middle age I followed the dictum that if you wanted a good tan you first had to get burned. It was often painful but ultimately very gratifying. In my twenties, once I had come out as a Gay man I realized how valuable a Speedo tan with a very sharp visible tan line could be beneficial for attracting other Gay men at the gym and pool. When I finally got the opportunity to vacation in Hawaii I realized that the sun exposure in the semi-tropical climate was even better for burning and tanning. My Hawaiian tan was deeper, darker and better than ever as was the sharp Speedo tan line. The burns were just as bad.

As I recounted earlier, I was more than likely first infected with the AIDS virus at the same time I was diagnosed with hepatitis in 1978. The presence of the AIDS virus and the AIDS cocktail predisposed me to be more susceptible to skin cancers than an ordinary sun worshiper. During the first couple of years following my AIDS diagnosis and in the first years in which I was covered by Kaiser Insurance I had several skin problems including episodes of actinic keratosis.

I began seeing Dr. Goldstein in my second year of AIDS diagnosis. As I recounted in an earlier chapter, I had had experiences with other Kaiser dermatologists and most of them were not particularly interested in listening to me or helping me with my dermatological problems. Since my friend and fellow AIDS patient, Walter Fernandes, told me about the comprehensive and compassionate new dermatologist, Dr. Goldstein, I made it my business to become his patient as soon as possible. It was probably one of the smartest decisions I had ever made.

Before my rapid decline in T-cells and my soaring viral load I was seeing Dr. Goldstein pretty regularly. I was always complaining about my sun-damaged scalp and the subsequent actinic keratosis and itching. It got so bad that at one point he sent me to his old UCSF mentor, Dr. Tim Burger. Burger was just as baffled by my itching as Goldstein had been. But once I went onto Hospice care my appointments with Dr. Goldstein declined. I think at one point the intervals between appointments were as much as six months.

Once I graduated from Hospice, as I told you before, I started to take the "AIDS cocktail" and my T-cells increased and my problems diminished, but by the middle of 2000 I was starting to have more skin problems. Yet I wasn't willing to face the music. Finally, shortly after the New Year I realized that I had to get back to see Dr. Goldstein. I complained to him about a strange skin anomaly on my right scalp. It was very red and bleeding.

Dr. Goldstein observed, numbed my scalp and took a biopsy. The biopsy of the lesion revealed an extensive squamous cancer. Dr. Goldstein scheduled an appointment for me with plastic surgeon, Dr. Ward.

In my appointment with Dr. Ward, he determined that I was a candidate for MOES surgery that would have to happen in an operating room under full anesthesia. That surgery is done in a special way because the process is designed to make sure all cancer is gone before suturing the wound. The surgeon begins by making a football shaped incision beyond what he perceives are the margins of the cancer. These marginal cuts are reviewed by a pathologist immediately after the extraction of the cancer. This extra pathology makes MOES surgery much lengthier than a simple removal. And one of the awful things that happened during this anesthetized procedure was that the anesthesia wore off and I regained consciousness. I was not happy. The anesthesiologist had to give me more anesthetic.

When the surgery was done and my wound bandaged, I discovered that because the wound was surrounded by hair the only way to bandage it was to wrap most of my head with gauze. These bandages were particularly daunting. I would not be able to bathe during the two weeks before the bandages would be removed and I would not be able to spend a lot of time in public.

Before I had the surgery I had scheduled a tour at the Frank Lloyd Wright Hexagon House on the campus of

Stanford University. It was going to be an excursion with my Most Holy Redeemer AIDS Support Group Volunteer. In addition we had invited my good friend Gary and a Welsh Catholic priest who was a correspondent for BBC Radio 4. The way I had met the Welsh priest was that while he was studying at the Jesuit School of Theology in Berkeley, he continued to do his human interest stories for the Welsh version of BBC Radio. Having investigated the Most Holy Redeemer AIDS Support Group, someone recommended that he interview me since I was an MHR parishioner and a support group client. On the day he did the interview, that would be broadcast to his Welsh listeners, Frank, my volunteer, and I were having our weekly meeting. When we told the priest about our excursion to Stanford he expressed an interest in joining us. So, several days after my dramatic surgery I joined these three other men with my head tightly wrapped in gauze. We all had a great time but I was highly embarrassed encased in a bandage that made me look like a mummy recently escaped from one of the pyramids.

I wish I could say that that was my last encounter with a scalpel. It wasn't; my skin cancer problems persist to the day I am writing this. From 2001 to 2007 my skin cancer surgeries seemed to occur on a regular periodic schedule, not close enough to each other to impact me seriously but still very annoying.

Then shortly after the big surgery and the big head covering bandage, Dr. Goldstein found another big squamous cancer on the opposite side of my forehead and scalp. Since I had established a good relationship with Dr. Ward, the surgeon who performed the first squamous cancer operation, I was glad he was going to be doing the next one. It had only been several months before that he had done the first cutting, nevertheless I had to go through it again.

Once this second surgery was done I was hoping I might have a break from further surgeries. That hope was not to be. Dr. Goldstein kept finding more and more skin cancers, some big, some infinitesimally small. They seemed to show up everywhere, on my face, near my eyes, on my ears, on every one of my limbs, and on my shoulders. As much as I hoped they would go away, they wouldn't. The damage had been done in my youth. The continual assault my immune system received from both the AIDS virus and the drugs that were addressing the various opportunistic infections I had faced or might face, profoundly affected my ability to fight the cancer that seemed unstoppable.

Chapter 15

Waiting for the

Other Shoe

To Drop

While dealing with all the skin problems caused by the cancers popping up all over my body, other problems were occurring. My T-cell count was better than the time before my Hospice experience when the sum total was a whopping ZERO and I had an AIDS viral load of 750,000. Before I transitioned to the first AIDS four drug "cocktail," the single drug therapy would raise my count to about 100 only to fall as the anti-retovirus mutated and the T-cells fell back to near zero. Then another single drug therapy produced the same result, etc.

Fortunately, when I switched to a four drug cocktail in early 1998, my T-cell numbers began to rise but hit an unexpected plateau. At the same time I was experiencing wild pendular swings with my blood sugars. My diabetes was totally out of control. Sometimes I would have a blood sugar reading of 500 or higher based on a scale where 100 is perfect and swings above or below this number were threatening my consciousness, my eyes and other organs, especially my kidneys. While high blood sugars are dangerous, lows can be deadly, and I was having a lot of lows, which frequently involved loss of consciousness, encounters with Emergency Medical Technicians, and rides to the Emergency Rooms, not to mention lectures from Diabetic Nurse Educators.

The fact is, I was still very angry about becoming a diabetic. After the pentamidine treatments destroyed my pancreas I was furious and became so uncooperative regarding my blood sugar stabilization that I was totally out of control. My anger resulted in completely failing to follow the advice of my medical practitioners. Since I had abstained from sugar for the eleven years before my diagnosis as a diabetic, I felt cheated. Before I started taking the new protease inhibitors I was simply a soon-to-die AIDS patient who happened to have diabetes; with the turn-around in my T-cells due to the protease inhibitors I became a diabetic who happened to have AIDS, now a seemingly survivable medical condition.

But there were many other things going on. I described the importance of a blood test called the Hemoglobin A1c. This test provides an index of blood sugar control over a period of three months. In the period after the introduction of the protease inhibitors my Hemoglobin A1c numbers were running about 10.0 or higher. My doctors and my Diabetic Nurse Educators knew I was lying about my diet but I didn't care. I still was angry and I wasn't worried about the consequences. One of the additional causes of these rises in Hemoglobin A1c was that the protease inhibitors also unbalanced the blood sugar issue. They made sugar control more difficult just as prednisone had.

One of the results of my lackadaisical attitude around blood sugar control, aside from my frequent hypoglycemic episodes usually resulting in serious losses of equilibrium, consciousness and other equally dangerous conditions, and other extreme problems, was the loss of hypoglycemic awareness. The normal human body has the natural ability to recognize when one's blood sugar has gone to low. Frequent episodes of low blood sugars cause this natural awareness to become less and less acute. Therefore, by the time one's blood sugar has fallen to much more dangerous lows extreme sweating commences and one has reached the point where the EMT's and emergency rooms become a regular part of one's life. All of these things began happening to me.

When these extreme events occur with regularity in the body of a diabetic other organs become involved. Probably the most vulnerable organs involved with out of control blood sugars are eyes and kidneys. The importance of eyes and vision is obvious; the kidneys' roles are less obvious. Aside from cleaning the blood and balancing the body's electrolytes, the kidneys also have a number of duties less well known. Among these functions is cooperating with the heart, particularly with regard to blood pressure. In addition the kidney is responsible for producing a hormone called erythropoietin. Erythropoietin is a hormone released to gather iron from the blood and then together to go to the bone marrow and produce new red blood cells.

The attack on my vulnerable organs dependent on good diabetic sugar control had begun to take its toll. The first sign of problems beyond blood sugar control was the escalating inability to control my blood pressure. Dr. Follansbee kept switching me from one blood pressure medicine to another. Sometimes he put me on more than one blood pressure medicine.

Several other unexpected medical crises followed. The first thing that happened was that my rising T-cells stopped rising. Simultaneously the ever important viral load, the test that measures how much of the HIV anti-retrovirus is present in the T-cells and how much they are replicating was rising higher. To get to the anti-retroviral cocktail that I was currently taking, many other drugs had been tried and found wanting. I told you about the story of the Sustiva disaster, but there were others. Some were not appropriate for diabetics. Some were harmful to the liver. Some caused extreme diarrhea. And some simply caused a terrible rash. Despite the plethora of new AIDS drugs coming onto the market, Dr. Follansbee felt that his hands were tied. At that point we had no other option but to stay the course with a limping failing cocktail. He literally said, "I have no other options." In some ways it felt like I was getting me ready to go back into Hospice. None of this news was good.

But that was not all. As my diabetes was getting more and more out of control, one of the very important functions of the kidney, the production of the hormone erythropoietin, had stopped. This stop had caused me to become more and more anemic. This was outside Dr. Follansbee's expertise of AIDS and infectious diseases. He admitted that he had no idea what to do. That my problems with blood pressure and anemia needed another set of eyes and he had just the man in mind.

Chapter 16

Doctor Yankulin

To the

Rescue

During the period between my Hospice graduation in 1998 and 2006, due to the introduction of a powerful AIDS cocktail, my T-cells began a remarkable rebound. Of course there was the scare caused by the mental problems associated with Sustiva. But fortunately that was handled deftly by Dr. Follansbee and a new drug substituted for the dangerous Sustiva. I was still having terrible problems with diarrhea, but eventually those were solved when we discovered that using dairy products at the same time as taking Norvir, one of the four drugs in my "AIDS cocktail," we found that it was the catalyst which triggered the diarrhea.

Unfortunately two unforeseen problems arose. First my T-cells suddenly hit a ceiling. They weren't rising the way they were in other patients. Dr. Follansbee was stymied and admitted to me that because of my allergies, diabetic problems, and alternative drugs' potential damage to other vital organs, he told me that we had run out of options. The second issue related to the inability to corral my blood pressures which were reaching dangerous levels, and the plummeting red blood cell counts which were being manifested by anemia and the loss of energy, enthusiasm and the ability to do almost anything. I was constantly exhausted.

Fortunately, Dr. Follansbee had enough self-esteem and honesty that he admitted that he had to turn me and my high blood pressure/anemia issues over to someone else.

At the same time my uncontrolled diabetes and astronomical Hemoglobin A1c's were of tremendous concern to both Dr. Follansbee and my extremely frustrated diabetic nurse educators. This also made it clear that re-enforcements were desperately needed.

For the diabetes, Dr. Follansbee and the Diabetic Nurse Educators kept begging me to begin using an insulin pump. Since the time when Dr. Celo, of UCSF and San Francisco General Hospital, had tried to get me to use an insulin pump to administer digestive enzymes hoping to help alleviate the extreme wasting syndrome to which I had been subjected as I entered Hospice care, I was very leery of those devices. That experience with the insulin pump to administer digestive enzymes was so painful that I simply demurred when anyone brought up the idea of using a pump. Instead of paying attention to the direness of my blood sugars and uncontrolled diabetes, I blithely continued to beat a path to destruction.

There is another test along with the A1c that is called the GFR, the glomular filtration rate. The GFR is an index of kidney function. My GFR was getting very bad with each blood test. A healthy GFR is around 60. By this point in my history, as Dr. Follansbee was desperately grasping for straws, my GFR was already in the 20's. And since I was ignorant about this test, it hardly fazed me. So in February 2007, Dr. Follansbee said, "There's this new young doc who's been having a lot of success turning around high blood pressure numbers, I'd like you to see him. His name is Dr. Yankulin." I have always been very leery of change and seeing Dr. Yankulin definitely qualified as change. But I thought, what could possibly go wrong. At least I'd see him once.

After Dr. Follansbee's referral, it took about two weeks to actually see Dr. Yankulin. Dr. Yankulin and I both have early Pisces birthdays, in fact a day apart, and we joked about that as that first appointment began. Like most referrals to specialists, [Dr. Yankulin is a kidney specialist known as a nephrologist], I expected this first appointment to last no more than fifteen or twenty minutes.

Once the polite greetings of patient and doctor were concluded, Dr. Yankulin revealed to me, for the first time, what an outstanding physician and diagnostician he is. He began by revealing how thoroughly he had reviewed, studied, and essentially memorized my medical history. I was astounded as I assented to each item he cited, convincing me that he was well aware of the challenges I had faced, and more astonishingly revealing most of what was going to happen to me.

Reviewing my blood pressure, anemia, and diabetic control issues, he gently but without mining any words told me that I was facing more than difficulties with high blood pressure and severe anemia. He then told me that within six months my kidneys would fail completely, I would have to go onto dialysis and that he would accompany me through all the stages leading to and receiving a kidney transplant.

At first I was simply dumbstruck. I knew things were not going well, but I hardly believed that things had gone this far. When I had turned the corner on my first life-threatening illness, AIDS, with the life-saving protease inhibitors, I hardly expected to be confronted by yet another frightening disease, one that had the words End Stage in its label. Kidney failure has the medical initials ESRD which stands for End Stage Renal Disease. These words mean that your body can definitely not take care of itself. And the "End Stage" part means you'll probably die if something drastic is not done immediately.

The only remedy for End Stage Renal Disease available other than a new, or should I say. previously owned kidney, is renal dialysis, and there are few medical procedures more onerous than dialysis. The ones that come to mind as being equally onerous are chemotherapy and radiation for cancer, but even those are limited in length. Once one starts dialysis, the only thing that stops it is a transplant, and sometimes that takes years, or death.

The reason that dialysis is so important is that once the kidney stops working several very bad things start happening. The kidneys have a number of important functions. They filter and balance the electrolytes in the blood. They provide a hormone responsible for assisting in the continual reproduction of red blood cells, and they help eliminate water absorbed from the colon by allowing us to urinate frequently. In some ways they are like a second brain or the body's department of balance. When the kidneys fail, when they stop working, everything goes out of balance. In the department of balance one of the unsuspected issues is the balancing of potassium. Potassium is one of the most important nutrients in many of our favorite foods, i.e., potatoes, tomatoes, oranges, avocados, and bananas. When one is in dialysis, one is forbidden to eat any of these foods. The reason is that eating these foods would counteract the dialysis process, increase the potassium making one's potassium dangerously high which then can impact the heart which can cause a massive heart attack, the expression is, "if your potassium is high you die."

At my first meeting with Dr. Yankulin I knew none of the above information. All I knew after my first visit with him is that I was in big trouble. He had told me that I would probably have to start dialysis within the next six months; that a kidney transplant would happen after I'd been on dialysis for a while; that he would schedule me for interviews at UCSF since Kaiser had been banned from doing transplants for some alleged improprieties; and that I would have to start having weekly injections of a drug that would artificially do what my kidneys were unable to do, produce the erythropoietin necessary for the production of red blood cells.

Almost in a daze after the many messages I had received from Dr. Yankulin, I scheduled my time for my first injection and headed home. I was very depressed but I knew I had a lot to tell Steve. I told Steve and he was expectedly as depressed as I was. After the hope that had been engendered by my bounce from the AIDS cocktail, this was one more example of how fragile my health really was.

I had many appointments following this first one with Dr. Yankulin. For one thing my AIDS cocktail was not working anymore and Dr. Follansbee had told me that he really didn't have any more drugs in his arsenal to help me. Either I had tried them and they had failed, or I was allergic to them or they had side effects that would either damage my liver or further compromise my already challenged kidneys. In addition, my uncontrolled diabetes had been one of the factors causing my End Stage Renal Disease. Until both of these conditions were remedied, I would definitely still require dialysis while my kidneys were still failing, but I would not be eligible for a lifesaving kidney transplants. End Stage Renal Disease would quickly lead to death. None of this was good news.

One of the unfortunate side effects of the weekly hormone injections was a rise in blood pressure. As Dr. Yankulin and Dr. Follansbee struggled to get my blood pressure under control, the hormone and my heightening blood pressure were working against me. Then, as my blood pressure continued to be more and more uncontrolled, it would stand as an obstacle to actually receiving the hormone shot, which once again exacerbated the anemia problem.

After a couple of weeks of hormone shots, my blood work showed little change in my red blood cell count. The anemia was not being remedied. The blood tests also showed that I didn't have enough iron in my blood to join with the injected hormone in order to create the new red blood cells. Dr. Yankulin's solution was to have me receive infusions of iron to assist the hormone in creating the red blood cells.

The key word was infusion, and the place to receive an infusion at Kaiser was the Infusion Center, the place where my AIDS journey had begun in 1993. So, when I got home from my appointment with Dr. Yankulin in the spring of 2007, I was surprised when I got a phone call from one of my former Infusion Center nurses, Iris. The first words from Iris were, "Frank Oliva? Is it really you?" Having seen me at my very worst, she was amazed that I was still alive. Nevertheless, she scheduled for a set of infusions to see if my red cell blood count could be increased.

The infusions actually worked but the continuing injections and blood pressure problems increased. By the middle of May, my blood pressure on occasion had reached the dangerously high 210/100, miles away from the new standard of 115/70. Once again I was in trouble.

These grotesquely high blood pressures were accompanied by extreme headaches, impossible indigestion and projectile vomiting. I couldn't even keep down water or Jell-O. A month later I went to my usual weekly hormone shot with a splitting headache, nausea and extremely high blood pressure. It was not the first time that I had a blood pressure too high to receive my hormone shot, but this time, not only did I not receive my shot but I was sent by ambulance to the Emergency Room.

I was triaged very quickly and Dr. Yankulin's presumptive diagnosis of a "hypertensive crisis" was confirmed. My condition involved galloping blood pressure, extreme nausea, and a splitting headache. After triage and evaluation, I was placed in TCU, one step down from ICU. The doctors prescribed reglan for nausea and a drug that must have been morphine, based on the fact that I became very dopey.

I spent the night in TCU and then was transferred to a private room for my convalescence and recovery. My nausea and headache had been treated. My blood pressure was restored to a more acceptable level and I began to receive guests. One of these guests was my newly acquired Diabetic Nurse Educator, Barbara Green. After much soul searching and counseling, Barbara had accomplished an amazing feat. She had turned around my miserable blood sugars. She was so effective that upon retirement she received a pay increase because of the turnaround. But Barbara knew that something much more permanent needed to be added.

On the day of my hypertensive crisis, an appointment with Barbara had been scheduled. The purpose of the appointment was to experiment with the dreaded insulin pump. It would inject saline rather than insulin to see if I could even tolerate the infusion set needed to support the insulin pump. Barbara came to my room after I was transferred from TCU and inserted the catheter to allow me to test the pump.

One of my very large problems with blood sugar control had to do with my very bad eating habits. Because of this I had been sent to a nutrition specialist. For the first time at Kaiser, I had met a nutritionist that I liked. Her compassion and moxie convinced me that I needed to make some changes. But when she heard about my hypertensive crisis she came to visit me. I told her how much I hated hospital food. She agreed with me and decided to go to Trader Joe's to smuggle me some edible food.

So, my hypertensive crisis, as bad as it was, had some silver linings. It was however a warning sign of something more malign like a stroke, but for the present I was to return to my normal activity. The following week I was back for my red blood cell hormone shot. Dr. Yankulin was very positive and told me that it was time to begin the process of exploring kidney transplant at UCSF.

UCSF has a much respected Kidney Transplant Program. The reason why Kaiser patients who need a kidney transplant have to go through UCSF to get a previously owned kidney is that Kaiser's fledgling Kidney Transplant Program ran into a dangerous legal problem the mechanics of which I really don't know or understand. After the controversy the solution was that Kaiser agreed that it would perform no more transplants, but instead funnel their transplant patients through the respected and tested UCSF program.

At Dr. Yankulin's suggestion, I attended the large group orientation at UCSF and then was seen by an individual counselor. First I learned that there were two pathways to transplant, one was to find a family member who had the same blood type and the willingness to donate his or her spare kidney. The other was that if a family member was not willing or able to donate a kidney, then my name would be entered on the list of those awaiting a kidney where I would have to reside for five to seven years. The other information that was given was the cost of a transplant operation and the cost of the medications I would need to take to keep the received kidney from being rejected. In the meeting with the pre-transplant coordinator I was also notified that there would be many more meetings and hurdles to be crossed before any operation would be scheduled.

I left my meetings at UCSF with hope, fear and doubt. The idea of replacing my failing kidneys was certainly hope for a life beyond end stage renal disease. The fears were many, among them were just the overall fear of surgery and all its risks, the fear of having to take more anti-rejection medicines necessary to prevent the transplanted kidney from being rejected, and the fear of the astronomical costs of the surgery and the new medicines. I knew I would have to make a decision but I really wasn't ready. Nevertheless, once I met with the UCSF personnel they began accruing my time on the waiting list.

Gradually, after my visit with UCSF administrators, I noticed that my anemic problems became considerably worse. Before my kidney failure became obvious in my blood work and my anemia started to diminish my energy, I had been a regular workout junkie. At first I just went to the gym to get out of the house. But as the protease inhibitors turned my T-cell count around and gave me much more enthusiasm in workouts, my attitude toward exercise grew as well. I eventually got to the point where I could stay on the stationary bike for almost two hours, and drench my gym clothes in sweat. As the kidney problems and anemia worsened my energy declined, eventually I had to stop working out altogether. I told Dr. Yankulin and he suggested that I just stop going to the gym for a while.

One of the things that became clear from the UCSF interviews is that I would not be eligible for a kidney transplant unless my T-cell count was improved and that brought us back to the dilemma that Dr. Follansbee had identified before he sent me to Dr. Yankulin. He didn't have any other drugs to replace the ones in my "AIDS Cocktail" that were no longer working. But by September three new drugs had become available. I was scheduled for an appointment at the Kaiser AIDS Research Clinic with my old friend, Brooke Anderson. I had first met Brooke when I participated in a UCSF CMV-retinitis drug study in

1994. Brooke was now the chief nurse administering many of the drug trials occurring at Kaiser.

One of the drugs in the potential replacement cocktail was a drug called Maraviroc or Selzentry. Unlike most AIDS cocktail drugs, this drug required a special test called a "tropic assay," something of which I had never heard before. A "tropic assay" is a test to determine whether or not the drug will be effective in terms of one's genetic conditions. Prior to these drugs I had had to submit to geno-typing and pheno-typing, essentially making sure that my version of the AIDS virus was not resistant to the drug being administered. But the tropic assay determined if my T-cells would be responsive to this new type of drug. Maraviroc had the ability to change intact CCR-5 markers to CCR-5 markers which were truncated. The reason that the truncated CCR-5 markers were so important because it had been discovered that intact CCR-5 markers were the easiest way for the AIDS virus to enter the T-cells where they could set up a "factory" for replication. It also was discovered that persons with truncated CCR-5 markers had inherited these markers from ancestors who had survived the Black Plague of the 14th Century. Obviously my ancestors were not Black Plague survivors; my CCR-5 markers were intact. I was a perfect candidate for AIDS infection and the "tropic assay" proved that I could be a very good candidate for the new drug.

Having passed the tropic assay, I began the new "AIDS Cocktail" on my spouse's birthday on September 26, 2007.

Meanwhile something unexpected happened. I had a friend of more than 20 years, who had moved to Berlin, Germany who used to call me from Berlin because he had an international calling plan. In one of those conversations, I asked him if he had been to Dresden to see the restored Frauenkirche. He responded that he hadn't because he had no one to join him on such a visit. Jokingly, I told him that I would be glad to join him but I couldn't afford the ticket to join him. He immediately offered to pay my air fare and to host me in his apartment.

All of a sudden I had the opportunity to travel to Berlin. The only obstacles were, would Steve consent to my travel and would Dr. Yankulin allow me to make the trip. Steve was reluctant to approve this rather risky trip but Dr. Yankulin endorsed it thinking that it would be spiritually beneficial for someone who was getting ready to enter the labyrinthine dialysis morass and its potential debilitating consequences.

With these approvals in place we set the travel dates. I flew to Chicago, changed planes for a flight to London with a connecting flight to Berlin which left on November 6, 2007. John was a wonderful host; I was able to see most of the important sites in Berlin, Leipzig, Dresden and Potsdam. I had some surprising reactions to my new "AIDS cocktail." I began to have an overwhelming odor of phosphorus. I especially felt like I smelled like laundry detergent.

I always have GI issues when I travel and this trip was not atypical. But I made a very big mistake on my last day. A friend of John's had invited me to join him for lunch at a Turkish restaurant. I have always been leery of exotic cuisines but I tried to be a good sport and I paid for this mistake in a very big way. My flight home was challenging and when I got home I felt awful.

I went as soon as possible to see Dr. Yankulin complaining of extreme GI pain. He examined me and then sent me for a CT scan. The diagnosis came back as diverticulosis, one more illness to be added to my ever-lengthening list. Dr. Yankulin was able to prescribe a medicine that remedied the diverticulitis. But once again it drove home to the doctors and me how much I needed to get ready for dialysis.

Then my malaise started manifesting in ordinary life. The way that I had to get back to Oakland after my San Francisco medical appointments was via AC Transit's Transbay buses. I remember one afternoon waiting for the P bus at the Transbay Terminal and feeling like I wasn't even going to able to get on the bus. I did, but when I got home I literally was ready to pass out.

Nevertheless, I kept trying to figure out ways to continually postpone the start of dialysis. One of the things that Dr. Yankulin almost insisted upon as a pathway to dialysis was that I get a fistula. Now a fistula is a very ambiguous word. One definition is a tear in the anus related to hemorrhoids; another definition is a large vein/artery which will remove the necessity of having an artificial catheter to allow the dialysis process. The vein/artery fistula requires an operation whereby a surgeon ties a vein to a nearby artery. What happens is that once joined, the fistula [the join of the vein and the artery] becomes large enough for the two very large gauge needles required for the cleansing of the blood which occurs during the dialysis.

Dr. Yankulin wanted my fistula operation to happen soon after my hypertensive crisis. I kept trying to postpone it. But something unexpected happened. Since 2001 I had had to have many skin cancer surgeries. One of the things I did not know is that the dirtier one's blood was the more reluctant the surgeons were to do skin cancer surgery, and my blood was at that point very dirty. As my anemia increased the tendency to develop skin cancers grew, and a big one had started to blossom on my left shin, and so when I went to see the surgeon to plan for the surgical removal of the shin skin cancer he said, "I will not operate until you have begun dialysis."

Suddenly my mind was made up. I could no longer delay dialysis, and by inference and implication, I knew I could no longer postpone my fistula surgery. In late November 2007 I saw the surgeon who would be doing my fistula operation. Since the fistula operation was essentially elective yet nonetheless critical, the surgeon had to find a time on the Operating Room schedule for the surgery to be done. We agreed on the scheduled time and did not get into the Operating Room until 10 PM.

As with any operation I was very nervous, but when Steve greeted me in the recovery room I was really glad that it was over. At that point you might think that the fistula operation was a done deal, unfortunately it wasn't. A fistula operation itself is not a done deal. It takes a couple of days for the "thrill" typical of the joining of a vein and an artery to be detectable, a much more obvious rapid pulse than the normal beat. To be palpable. When the surgeon saw me several days after the surgery he realized that the expected thrill was not present, that essentially the fistula surgery had been a failure and he decided to do another surgery. I asked that it be postponed until after Christmas.

The next fistula surgery happened in mid-January and the same thing happened. Because I was born right-handed it was decided that I should have my fistula in my left arm. But it was discovered that because of the many infusions I had had for pneumocystis and CMV retinitis many of the superficial veins in my left arm had been blown and since the objective of creating a fistula is to allow the circulation of blood in and out of the arm required by dialysis, this was critical. Unfortunately, these blown veins did not allow the fistula to be created. And so a third operation was required.

By the time the third operation was scheduled, I was a lot closer to the point where dialysis was necessary. Steve had been available to take me home after the first two operations, but after three months without work Steve had been hired unexpectedly by PG&E and his first day at work was the day of my third fistula operation. At this point my blood pressure was also dangerously uncontrolled. My friend Rob, who had been helping me with our rooftop garden and our dog, was able to take me to Kaiser for the surgery. He also would remain with me until Steve arrived after his first day at his new job.

This operation happened on time. This time the surgeon tied a vein and artery together in the bend in my right arm. Since I always require so much anesthesia to be appropriately unconscious for the operation, it also takes a lot longer for me to recover. I don't know if what happened after the surgery was related to my hypertensive crisis eight months earlier, but as I remained unconscious after the surgery my blood pressure spiked dangerously high. And while I was unconscious, the nurses in the recovery room were basically ignoring me.

Fortunately, my good friend, Rob King was attending me and becoming more and more concerned as my blood pressure rose. Finally, he had had enough of watching me in what appeared to him to be another crisis. He summoned the courage to alert the nurses who were ignoring me, to start paying attention. This call to attention got the nurses to call Dr. Yankulin who arrived within minutes. He assessed the situation and prescribed immediately an injection of clonidine to assist in lowering my blood pressure and by the time Steve arrived after his first day at his new job, my blood pressure had been lowered to an acceptable number. I got dressed, said goodbye to Dr. Yankulin and headed home.

I was exhausted after this third surgery to create a fistula for dialysis. And, because I needed so much IV fluid since I always require more anesthesia than other patients, my body had more fluid in it and created a very unbalanced system. The surgery happened on February 27th. I spent the following day alone while Steve was at his new job, doing nothing but resting. I recuperated for the rest of the weekend dealing with the exhaustion caused by the surgery and the out of control blood pressure. I was having difficulty eliminating the excess fluid both because of my failing kidneys and my lack of activity. I had been troubled with continuing anemia despite my injections. What happened when I had too much fluid in my body is that my ankles swelled uncomfortably, which in medical terms is called edema.

On Monday nights for the past several years I had been meeting with one of my sponsees and Monday March 3rd was no different. But this Monday was significantly different from the others because the edema had gone to my lungs, and this is termed congestive heart failure which is a very debilitating condition, and also life threatening. And the way this particular congestive heart failure was affecting me is that I could barely speak because breathing had been so difficult. I tried conducting this session while resting on a couch but even that became too difficult.

Even after leaving San Francisco I did not transfer my health care to Oakland. But this experience of congestive heart failure forced me to terminate my meeting with my sponsee and ask Steve to take me to the Kaiser Oakland Emergency Room. The bad news is that I was treated much more peremptorily by the ER staff in Oakland than I had ever been in San Francisco. I felt like I was not being treated in the most professional manner and it really put me in a worse mood than the one in which I had arrived.

Eventually it was determined that I needed to be admitted. I was glad until I got to my room. For years Kaiser Oakland, realizing that they desperately needed to build a new hospital with better rooms, had been stonewalled by the city of Oakland to the point that Kaiser Oakland threatened to move to Emeryville if the hospital's new construction was not approved. Kaiser's alternate planning convinced Oakland authorities that the proposed move would be very bad for Oakland and they relented. But the new hospital was still on the drawing board and on this night of desperately needing to be admitted to a room, I think I was given the worst bed in the worst room in the extremely overcrowded hospital.

I was already miserable considering how the congestive heart failure had deflated me. But my misery was increased exponentially when I discovered that one of the men in my over-crowded three bed hospital room was an older angry African American who immediately told me which bathroom I could use. My discomfort became acute. Fortunately, somewhere in the middle of the morning, Dr. Yankulin called me and told me that the Oakland nephrologist was a friendly colleague of his and would take care of me. Shortly after Yankulin's phone call, the Oakland nephrologist visited me and told me that he thought I needed to start dialysis. Since my fistula was less than five days old, there was no way it was mature enough to use for dialysis; the only alternative was an emergency surgery to create a port and then dialyze me.

Now I was truly terrified. The reason why I was experiencing this congestive heart failure experience was because my kidneys had not been able to clear the fluid for which the fistula was needed and now the nephrologist wanted to do another surgery. I immediately contacted Dr. Yankulin and begged him to halt all the nightmares being proposed for me. Fortunately, he suggested Lasix as a way to lower the excess fluid that caused the congestive heart failure and I dodged another bullet.

By the grace of God I was released the next day and went home to another convalescence following both the fistula surgery of the previous week and the congestive heart failure that followed it on Monday.

I knew dialysis was on the way. I knew how bad my anemia had gotten. I really began to fear for my survival. A fistula takes at least six weeks to bulk up to be ready for dialysis. By my calculation, that meant the middle of April. I dragged myself through March having staggeringly high blood pressures. I was exhausted all the time. Easter in 2008 was on March 23rd. So by mid-April it was far in my rearview mirror.

Once I make up my mind it is pretty hard for anyone to change it. Dr. Yankulin knew that dialysis for me was not too far in the future, but he tried to postpone it. He didn't think my fistula was ready. With an undeveloped fistula it is more difficult to insert the needles. The less developed the fistula the smaller the gauge of the needles used which makes the flow that much slower, resulting in more pain. I had no idea what was coming but I was insistent.

Because dialysis usually is done three times a week for at least three hours plus a half hour prep and a half hour clean up, Dr. Yankulin felt it would be better for me to have my dialysis in Oakland because of the time involved, but he would supervise the first one in the Hemodialysis Clinic in the San Francisco Kaiser Hospital. The start date was set for April 16th.

Before my first dialysis my friend Michael decided that I needed a special treat. He took me to the Tartine Bakery on 16th Street to have the incredibly delicious and fat-loaded bread pudding, despite my diabetes. After consuming the bread pudding I took the bus to Kaiser expecting my first dialysis to begin before noon. As usual the Hemodialysis Unit had a more flexible version of a schedule, not the Mussolini Train Schedule I expected. I was told my time would not come until 1 PM or 1:30, so I did something really stupid. In a self-indulgent moment I decided I needed another treat.

There is a fast-food restaurant up the street from Kaiser's Hospital on the opposite side of the street. It is just one point above a "greasy-spoon." It serves real "comfort food," that is, greasy cheese burgers, greasy fries, and carbo-loaded milkshakes. What could possibly go wrong?

Despite my diabetes and the relatively close time of my FIRST dialysis, I indulged in this very dangerous lunch. It was a short walk across the street to my check-in and the first dreaded placement of the dialysis needles. Needless to say, my blood pressure was high and my stomach was growling from my injudicious lunch.

Before the dialysis actually began with the placement of the needles, there was a lot of paperwork. And since Dr. Yankulin had determined that once I started dialysis I would transition to a larger dialysis for-profit center in Oakland which would be more practical and efficient despite the fact that it would remove me from Dr. Yankulin's direct care, dialysis in San Francisco would only last a week.

Chapter 17

Dialysis Begins

It had finally happened. Dr. Yankulin had predicted in February 2007 that I would have to have dialysis in six months. Fourteen months had elapsed since that prediction. On April 16, 2008, after my very greasy and very inappropriate lunch I entered the Hemodialysis Center on the first floor of Kaiser San Francisco Hospital. I had been there a little more than an hour but this time I was met by Dr. Yankulin, the charge nurse, and the nurse who would be inserting the needles in my less than mature fistula.

I was shown to my bed with its television and dialyzer where I would spend the next three to four hours. I took off my shoes and got on the bed and with a queasy stomach, a nervous mind and heavy heart prepared for yet another unknown.

Of course the most terrifying things were the frightening needles, and despite all the forms and paperwork and signatures, they paled next to the needles. A charming nurse approached me reassuringly and told me it was time. She thoroughly disinfected the place on my fistula where she would insert the needles, one connected to the line leading to the dialyzer with my soiled blood, the other returning the blood that had been cleansed.

Lidocaine always preceded the insertion of the needles but it did little to arrest the pain on the first insertion. And this was only the beginning, who knew how long this process would last. I knew this dialysis would be over in about three hours, but it would happen two days after this and two days after that until such time as I received someone else's kidney. Would that be in less than five years or sooner? No one had any idea, only that the dialysis journey had begun.

The queasiness, with which I began this first dialysis, caused by an incredibly inappropriate lunch, morphed into full blown nausea. I was unable to complete the three hours of a typical dialysis, and then when I stood up from my dialysis I immediately threw up most of my lunch.

After recovering from my embarrassment, I adjusted my clothes, put on my shoes and met my cousin, Veronica, who had volunteered to drive me back to Oakland. Unsteadily, I walked with her to her car. As I got into the car, another wave of nausea hit me, but I was able to suppress the need to vomit. I hoped I would make it home before it hit again. But I couldn't; after we'd driven the streets leading to the Bay Bridge everything changed. Suddenly I could no longer suppress the urge to vomit, and most of what was left in my agitated stomach was heaved into Veronica's car. The damage wasn't great, but again, it was this terribly embarrassing thing of vomiting in someone else's car.

Once I got home I thought I would collapse completely and I ruminated about the possibility of doing this three times a week until I would be eligible to receive someone else's kidney. If I chose the ordinary transplant track it would be a minimum of five years before I would become eligible for a transplant unless I found a family member donor. And this I had chosen never to do because I did not want to put anyone through this process. The other option was to be placed on the high-risk donor list which was purported to be a much faster though riskier list.

But meanwhile I had survived my first dialysis and was dreading the next one, two days later. It was no longer a mystery; I now knew how much pain and misery was involved in this process. I was extremely depressed but on the next day I summoned the courage and energy to make it to my second dialysis appointment. The second dialysis was less of a trial than the first had been, and much of the dialysis time was spent figuring out where I would have dialysis once I transitioned to an Oakland dialysis facility. The one selected was relatively close to my home and would reduce the commute significantly. It would also involve transitioning away from Dr. Yankulin and San Francisco Kaiser and entering the care of the nephrologist who had wanted to create an emergency port for dialysis when I had had the congestive heart failure episode after my fistula operation.

My first day at RAI Dialysis Center was frightening. The small Hemodialysis Clinic at Kaiser's Hospital in San Francisco has only eight dialysis stations. The Oakland RAI Dialysis facility looked like a factory. As I recall, there were about ninety chairs divided into three sections of thirty. Each section was served by about five technicians of varying skill sets, each being supervised by two nurses. Since the facility served patients from several Oakland hospitals, each hospital provided its own nephrologist who visited intermittently; the Kaiser doctor visited once every three or four weeks. In the Kaiser Hemodialysis Center, at least one doctor was on duty several times each day.

The first couple of treatments were very uncomfortable and I wasn't able to be dialyzed for the full three hours. This was neither good news for me nor for my kidneys. Then something really terrible happened.

As I said in my introduction of my time at the RAI Dialysis Center, the skill of those technicians placing the needles in the patients' fistulas varied from excellent to abysmal. The first three technicians were adequate though not great. The fourth on was quite inexperienced. Since my fistula was about two months old and no fistula could be used until it was at least six weeks old, it was certainly very fragile.

When this less than experienced technician inserted the needles she was not very careful and one of the needles pierced the fistula wall causing infiltration of blood into my muscle and unbearable pain. I was unable to be dialyzed that day. The pain did not stop after the needles were removed. It lasted all weekend and upset me, my spouse and Dr. Yankulin.

The apologies were profuse. The Dialysis Center begged me to come back and promised me that this would never happen again. The reality is that once one has started dialysis the danger of interrupting it is frightening. Usually, after stopping dialysis for a week, death is almost always the result.

Although my initial reaction was to stop going to this clinic which had injured me grievously, I knew that I could not stop dialysis without putting my life in imminent danger. On Monday I reluctantly returned to RAI. I was given a much more experienced technician and the dialysis proceeded with no particularly noticeable consequence. It turned out that I had two dependable technicians; one was a young African American man who was very deft in placing the smallest gaged needles. There also was a Hispanic middle-aged woman technician who was equally experienced.

In the middle of the following month I chose to attend a San Francisco Symphony morning rehearsal. As I approached the Symphony Hall in San Francisco's Civic Center, I noticed an unusual number of press and television vans in front of the Supreme Court of the State of California. I called Steve at work and asked him if he knew what was going on. He told me that the Supreme Court of California was set to rule on the question of same-sex marriage. I rolled my eyes and expressed doubt and told him I would call at intermission to hear the actual ruling.

The concert rehearsal was fantastic. Los Angeles Philharmonic's *wunderkind*, Gustavo Dudamel, gave a stupendous reading of Stravinsky's *Rite of Spring*. At intermission I called Steve and he floored me when he said that the Supreme Court of California had ruled that any law against same-sex marriage was unconstitutional and that Gay marriages would begin being performed as early as June 15th. I immediately asked Steve if he would marry me and as quickly he said yes. I left the very satisfying concert on cloud nine. But the next day it would be back to dialysis.

While I was sequestered to Kaiser Oakland, Dr. Yankulin had arranged an appointment with an Oakland cardiologist. After about a month of dialysis I went to the appointment with the Oakland Kaiser cardiologist. The reason why this appointment was so important is that one of the gateways to kidney transplant was a procedure known as cardiac catherization. Cardiac catherization involves inserting a line into the femoral artery, the large artery that serves the leg and begins in the groin right below the testicles. Once this line is placed, the catheter includes a camera; this line is then threaded up into the heart and the aorta, to determine whether or not the heart will be able to endure the rigors of a kidney transplant. Hence this procedure is the make or break gatekeeper to become eligible for a kidney transplant.

You can imagine how anxiously and hopefully I entered the cardiologist's office. Then moments after the discussion began, my hopes were dashed to pieces. The cardiologist told me there was no way my heart would be healthy enough to endure the cardiac catheritization, let alone a kidney transplant. Since I knew that my days were definitely numbered if I did not get a transplanted kidney I left the appointment with a feeling that I was going to die and shortly.

I went to my next dialysis appointment with a "why bother" attitude. I felt my situation was truly hopeless. Nevertheless, I looked forward to our wedding and we planned a special getaway weekend in Carmel. A friend of mine had told me about Doris Day's dog friendly hotel in Carmel. It was very expensive but it seemed like an ideal treat for a family that had been reeling after the challenges of a month and a half of dialysis. I had to make special arrangements with RAI to allow this extended weekend to happen. They allowed me to have dialysis on Friday morning before we left, and Monday afternoon after we had returned from Carmel. The weekend was wonderful but once we were back my extreme depression was again overwhelming me.

But we still had the wedding to plan and in the middle of June Steve and I purchased some wonderful ties at Macy's. We notified a few friends and asked them to join us on July 22nd at San Francisco's City Hall. These feelings of hope buoyed me as I tried to forget that I was not being allowed a cardiac catheritization which would, in turn, prevent me from getting a transplanted kidney.

It's hard to tell which crisis precipitated me to the next disaster. I continued to go to my regular dialysis appointments after the disappointing news regarding the cardiac catheritization and the death sentence it imposed on me. I looked forward to our wedding and I tried to forget about the problems I was facing.

I had discovered that it wasn't that hard to walk to and from dialysis. I would walk Bo, skip lunch and leave the house around 12:30 PM for a 1 PM dialysis appointment. The needles still hurt but my excellent technicians were able to minimize the pain. I actually succeeded in enduring the full three hours without having to terminate the session because I was in too much pain.

Then, in late June during an extraordinary heat wave where we experienced temperatures of 100° at midnight that forced Steve, me and Bo to try to sleep on our deck because our bedroom was too stifling. We got no sleep that Friday night because there was a very full June moon.

In the extreme heat that continued to plague us, I set out for Monday's dialysis trying to brave the temperature. I was on time for my treatment, and settled quickly in my chair, but then something completely unexpected and unanticipated happened. Unlike the previous dialysis days following the infiltration disaster of late April, both of my favored technicians had taken a Monday holiday.

I was both angry and terrified. I didn't know what to do. While waiting, one of the nurses, supervising the technicians in my section of the facility, approached me. She told me, in a less than a compassionate way that I had to be open to having my dialysis started by technicians other than my favorites. I was furious. I seriously thought of just walking out and skipping my dialysis session, but in spite of myself I decided to go through with it.

When it was over I left in absolute fury. I don't remember but I'm sure my blood pressure was sky high. I didn't care. I stormed out of RAI and vigorously strode up the hill despite the heat, despite my lack of composure simply raging about the facility and the way I had been treated by that condescending nurse.

When I got home, I waited for Steve to arrive from work. We had dinner and I tried to have a normal evening but I was still seething. When it came time to go to bed, I was way too agitated to go to sleep.

I had been way too upset so I decided to watch a DVD of Dickens' *Nicholas Nickelby.* But by 11:45 I felt that I really needed to go to bed. However, when I got to the top of the stairs to descend to our bedroom, a wave of dizziness hit me, I stumbled, my blood pressure was way too high to get to sleep. I turned around and sat down to watch the rest of *Nicholas Nickelby.* Once it ended at about 2:30 AM I decided to try going to bed again. Somewhat wobbly I descended the stairs and succeeded in getting into bed but I still had a very hard time getting to sleep. Then it happened, in spite of a completely darkened room I saw a bright blue flash of light followed by the tinkling sound of breaking glass. "What was that?" I said to myself, trying to ignore what had just happened. I really wanted to get to sleep, but I couldn't. I was too frightened. As my body started to stiffen, I thought about trying to awaken Steve but I was stopped by the feeling that he needed his sleep and whatever had happened could keep until morning.

Chapter 18

All Strokes Are

Unexpected

This One

Surely Was

So the blue light in a completely darkened room followed by the eerie sound of breaking glass had happened. It was about 2:45 AM and I had decided to let Steve sleep. He had to get up at 5:30 so I figured he might as well sleep. As I lay in bed, I kept thinking, "I wonder if that was a big stroke, bigger than the little one I had had before I returned to the study to finish my movie."

In spite of these thoughts I still tried to get to sleep, but my blood pressure and my fear kept me awake. Finally, around 5:00 AM, after feeling my body stiffen for the past two hours, I woke Steve and told him I thought I had had a stroke. He was in shock but he went into action. While he rushed to get dressed and take Bo out to pee so he could then focus on me, I struggled to get out of bed and fell to the floor.

Since our bedroom is on a floor below the main body of the apartment, after struggling to get dressed, I had to attempt to crawl up the stairs with my working left side. The stroke had paralyzed my right side. Once I got to the top of the stairs, Steve brought a rolling chair from the computer room and rolled me to the elevator in order to steer me toward the car.

Since moving from San Francisco to Oakland I had kept my primary care in San Francisco's Kaiser. I hated Oakland Kaiser, particularly after my terrible experience in March with congestive heart failure; I vowed that I would never enter Kaiser's Oakland facility again. Therefore calling an ambulance was completely out of the question. I insisted that Steve drive me to the Emergency Room at San Francisco's Kaiser Hospital on Geary Boulevard.

Fortunately, it was early enough that the Bay Bridge was very quiet. We made it to the hospital in record time. When we got there Steve asked the team on duty to bring a wheel chair for me since I had had a pretty significant stroke and had lost the use of my right side.

I had never been triaged so quickly. I was whisked into a private room, something very different from my previous visits to the Emergency Room. They were extremely attentive. I was immediately sent for a CT scan and as I was wheeled on the gurney for this test I saw Dr. Yankulin passing through the hall. I was so glad to see him; it made me much more at peace.

While I was having the CT scan, Steve called my parents to tell them what had happened. They were in shock. When I got back to the room I got a chance to speak to them, but already my speech was showing signs of difficulty. The right side of my mouth could not keep up with the unaffected left.

After numerous rechecks and evaluations I was admitted to a room on the stroke floor. The seventh floor is a very interesting floor. The last time I had been housed on this floor was after the hypertensive crisis of 2007. My room had been very close to the nurses station and by the time I left I was so sick of the nurses' call signal, which was a computer manufactured rendition of the children's nursery rhyme, "Mary had a little lamb," that if I never hear it again, it will be way too soon. This time, my room was as far away from the dreaded nurses' station as possible; it was just fine with me.

By the time I got to my room it was very close to bed time. Steve had stayed with me as long as possible, but he had to get home to our dog, Bo. Alone and in a hospital room with so many LED lights on numerous pieces of equipment including a blood pressure cuff that seemed to be programmed to take my blood pressure every fifteen minutes, it was virtually impossible to get to sleep despite the fact that my last moments of sleep were on Sunday night. At that point I was trying to fall asleep after forty-eight hours of being awake. But that was not the only thing keeping me awake. In January 1964, my maternal grandmother had died from a major stroke due to hardening of the arteries. My thoughts were, "Is that what is happening to me?" I tossed and turned in fear and sadness. I thought of my grandmother who I had loved so much. And, as if all this wasn't enough, the nurses and medical assistants on duty frequently entered the room lighting all the lights and torturing my eyes that had not been dilating very well because of blood pressure problems.

When the sun rose, I was glad that my tossing and turning could stop. At least I could now be legitimately awake. All of my doctors visited me in my room. Steve stopped by to visit before he went to his job at PG&E. In the middle of the morning, my friend Walter, who had been a member of our Most Holy Redeemer AIDS Support Group stopped by to visit me. I was very glad to see him, but the most interesting news he brought me was about a book by a stroke survivor, Jill Bolte Taylor. He told me about her amazing book, *My Stroke of Insight*. He told me that the book detailed mental recovery of brain power through meditation on the right side of the brain. I was still reeling from the brain attack I had just had, but this seemed like a resource to aid my recovery. The night before I had questioned whether there would be any recovery but with this message on this June morning at least I had a glimmer of hope.

The next surprise was the first visit from a physical therapist. In spite of the fact that my stroke had happened a little more than thirty-six hours before, my therapy was beginning. She actually got me out of bed to try and walk with a quad cane. I was amazed. I'm not sure if I ever expected to walk again or be able to do anything. She was filled with enthusiasm and hope. I was shocked. Anything she asked me to do was very hard, but she was so encouraging that I tried in spite of myself.

Believe it or not she actually had me stumbling with the quad cane. It was tremendously exhausting and the exercises came to an end.

The remaining days of hospitalization were occupied with daily rehabilitation, dialysis, and daily observation by all my doctors, plus a very vigorous discussion of where I might go for further rehabilitation, my home was clearly not an option.

One of the things that would need to be in place was the convenience of receiving dialysis every other day. This dialysis requirement obviated many of the available facilities and made one much more desirable than the others. This most desirable facility was Kaiser's own Vallejo Rehabilitation Hospital, affectionately known as KFRC. This designation stood for Kaiser Foundation Rehabilitation Center. Its acronym was particularly amusing to persons of my age. It had been probably the most popular "teen" radio station in the San Francisco Area when I was a teen. KFRC was the facility that Dr. Yankulin was most anxious to have me enter.

But there were many obstacles to admission. KFRC was the most coveted stroke rehabilitation site in all of northern California's Kaiser Service area, and therefore it was very difficult to be admitted there. The ironic thing is that the physical therapists told me that I could not make too much progress in San Francisco or I would not be admitted to the Vallejo facility. There also was the issue of bed availability, and until that was ready I would not be able to be moved.

During my stay in the hospital, my parents visited me. It was a very uncomfortable meeting. Then my sister, brother and my sister's husband visited me. My brother said one of the most amusing and remarkable things to me. He said, "This is nothing like a usual hospital visit, it is way too much fun." There was a lot of laughter and it really did a lot to cheer me.

I had had my stroke early on a Tuesday morning. A weeklong hospital stay was more than most Kaiser patients are afforded. And by the following Tuesday it was time for me to go. But after a week in the hospital mostly confined to my bed and unable to bathe without assistance I needed a shower. Steve offered to assist me in the hospital shower and the nurses gave their consent.

Well we were hardly ready for this experience. Steve tried his best, but my footing was so unsure and my ability to remain standing so inadequate that I fell several times in the shower. But once Steve and I felt I had been sufficiently scrubbed, he assisted me getting out of the shower, dried and dressed me so that I was ready for transport to Vallejo Kaiser's KFRC.

Chapter 19

KFRC

Once I was dressed and ready to make the trip to Vallejo, I had to wait for the ambulance that would transport me. The only way Kaiser Hospital would allow me to be transported to KFRC was by paramedics in an ambulance with all the necessary vital-sign monitors attached.

The paramedics transported me on a gurney turned into a wheelchair onto the elevator to ride from the 7th floor to the ambulance entrance of the Emergency Room. Steve, meanwhile, went to our car. He would try to follow the ambulance over the Bay Bridge and up I-80 to Vallejo. I was loaded into the ambulance and we traveled at normal speed onto the city streets heading for the bridge. We were too fast for Steve and he had to find his way to Vallejo without benefit of maps, GPS, which we did not have at the time, or any sense of where the facility was. And he remained too slow to follow directly behind the ambulance.

The ride across the Bay Bridge was very strange. After a week on the Stroke floor of Kaiser Hospital this was a journey which I would have preferred to take in our CRV, Steve at the wheel and me so excited at the prospect of going home and seeing our dog, Bo. But that was not to be. I was facing backwards on the gurney in the ambulance going to a place I had never been before, with no idea what would happen or how long I would have to stay at KFRC, Vallejo.

Eventually we arrived at the Kaiser Vallejo Hospital in its dedicated state-of-the-art rehabilitation facility nicknamed "KFRC." The EMT's off-loaded me from the ambulance and wheeled me into the facility up to the admission desk. But it was noon and everyone was at lunch. I was stuck on a gurney in a hallway outside the registration area, left like a UPS package by a driver who had found that no one was home.

During that "warehouse" experience, Steve called me to tell me that he had no idea how to find the facility. Fortunately, just before Steve had called me, Wanda, the charge nurse, returned. I gave her my cell phone and she was able to give Steve directions to the facility. And, I was somewhat concerned about Steve's arrival, because not only did I want to see him, but also, he had purchased all the required items I would need during my stay at KFRC. Anecdotally, KFRC had given us a list of the things I would have to bring, not unlike a list of items a kid needs to bring to summer camp.

When Steve arrived Wanda showed us to my four man room or ward. I had never had to stay in such a hospital ward. This did not make me happy. As Steve and I waited for the intake staff to arrive and acquaint us with what my stay would involve, we met the cast of characters who would be my roommates for at least part of my stay. There was a man in the bed opposite mine who was in the facility for a very unusual disease that seemed to cause muscle degeneration. During the course of my stay, we had many friendly conversations, and he became my closest "friend" in the facility. Kitty-corner to me was a very young man who had been in a serious motorcycle accident, and he was so disruptive that his bed had to be covered with a cage that reminded me of one of those inflatable kid-party houses. The man next to me was the one with whom I had the least interaction. He was much older than the rest of us and rarely had his confidentiality curtains open. The interesting thing is that he too was a diabetic dialysis patient who had had a stroke. He had the most similar case to mine but we never interacted.

Then the representatives of the actual rehabilitation staff came to talk to Steve and me. Since my speech had been affected by the stroke, Steve did most of the talking. The staff representatives presented me with quite a bit of information. First of all, they would have to accommodate my three times a week dialysis into my rehabilitation schedule. After all, one of the reasons for selecting KFRC was because of the on campus dialysis facility. During the conversation the most important issues discussed were my rehab goals. Not missing a beat, Steve told the staff members that we had scheduled our marriage ceremony for Tuesday, July 22nd, a mere three weeks away. The staff immediately made that one of my rehab goals. In addition there were the goals of regaining as much physical function that the stroke had taken and of trying to combat the very depressing mood which had descended on me. The functions that I had lost, perhaps temporarily, perhaps permanently, were articulate speech, the ability to walk unaided, the ability to use most of my right side, including my right hand, and the ability to close my right eye and the right side of my mouth.

The intake team assured me that each of these disabilities would be addressed and that I should have most of these faculties restored to me. I was hopeful but skeptical. They encouraged both Steve and me that they had a state-of-the-art rehabilitation facility with international fame and international therapists. During the intake they measured me for a wheel chair which would be my principle means of movement for the duration of my stay.

We also met the other professionals who would be participating in my care, including a social worker, a patient ombudsman, and a psychotherapist.

Eventually it became time for Steve to return to our home in Oakland and take care of our dog, Bo, who had been alone since the morning hours and needed his midday walk and his dinner. It was going to be a trying time for all of us.

After Steve left, I reclined on my bed and began getting to know the roommate with whom I had the most in common. We told each other a little bit of our medical histories and the disabling events that had brought us to KFRC. We both looked at each other with somewhat hopeless wry smiles. He may have thought I had more likelihood of success than he had. My case had to do with manageable medical issues; his problems had more to do with genetics.

Then something really unexpected happened. Steve had dressed me in the loose, almost sweat pants like pants, required attire for patients in this facility, they were very comfortable. The guy, who came to see me, said that he needed to measure my arms and legs. No one had ever asked me for this before. He had to remove my pants; he had closed my privacy curtains. He did the measurements and then told me that this would be happening every day.

When the measurer left, the woman who would be my nurse arrived. I was somewhat skeptical about her, but I tried to put a good face on it. So far this facility had been unlike any in which I had been treated. They were much more observant and attentive than any other hospital personnel I had encountered.

Not long after, another technician came to tell me that dinner would be served soon and that I would have to test my blood sugar and pre-emptively dose for what was going to be served to me. This became one of the banes of my existence during my stay at KFRC. I have always been one of the most finicky eaters in the world. If I don't like it, or like the look of it, or like the smell of it, or I don't like the name of it, I won't even consider eating it. This posed a very dangerous problem. If one gives an insulin dose for a certain number of carbohydrates and doesn't consume said carbohydrates the results can be disastrous, and this became a common occurrence. The terrible results did not happen immediately, but usually after I had fallen asleep. Hypoglycemia is one of the most dangerous conditions a diabetic can face, because if left unattended, the insulin-overdosed diabetic can proceed into a coma followed by death.

This was one of the reasons it was good that I was placed in a ward rather than a private room. One of the things that annoyed me about the patient immediately on my right was that his wife was not only hovering over him, she was actually sleeping in the room with him and us. I felt this was a gross violation of the rights of the four men in the room, and I am quite sure that if a husband had decided to stay in a women's room with his wife, the women would have demanded that he be removed. But it actually turned to be lucky that she was so close to me. Her husband's condition was very much like mine despite the fact that he was so much older than I, and when I displayed in my sleep the behavior she had seen so often in her diabetic husband, she immediately alerted the night nurse and she administered the necessary glucose to prevent me from proceeding, to death.

The day after my intake was a dialysis day. I had been dialyzed in San Francisco the day before my transfer, so my first day of classes would be punctuated by my first dialysis at Kaiser Vallejo. This day was also my first day of classes and my first class was called Occupational Therapy, distinguished from Physical Therapy; simply put Occupational Therapy deals with the thing one does with one's hands like eating and self-care, Physical Therapy on the other hand deals with movement, and in addition I had to learn how to navigate my wheelchair. Since I no longer had the use of my right hand or right foot, I had to learn to use my weak left hand, (I was born right-handed) and my weak left foot to move forward in the wheelchair. I had to use my left hand to power the wheel of the chair and use my left foot to steer. Believe me, this was a tremendous challenge.

During this first class, that was really one on one tutoring, I had to plunge my right hand into a bucket of ice and hot water. I tried to do the exercises that the therapist wanted me to do but this was extremely difficult.

Once the Occupational Therapy concluded after an hour of torture, I was very glad to proceed to Speech Therapy. The muscles around the mouth are very different from the rest of the body. They are circular, but a left brain stroke directly impacts the right side of the mouth muscles. As time passed, my affected muscles became stiffer by the day. At this point my stroke had happened more than a week before. The two sides of my mouth were not co-operating with each other. The left wanted to talk as quickly as my excited brain. The stroke affected right side simply could not keep up. Therefore, throughout my stay, my Speech Therapist continually exhorted me to slow down my left side so that the right could catch up.

Following my first two tutorials, which were in very small rooms, my next class was in the large gym. The first class was Gait, and this one also involved a private tutor. This tutorial addressed my need to relearn walking. Finally I got to get out of my wheelchair. This tutorial involved a lot of floor exercise and my first attempt to walk assisted by parallel bars where I was taught to put one foot in front of another. If the first classes were difficult, this one was almost impossible.

When the first class in the gym ended the next one was in another section of the same gym, and this one was as a participant with ten or so other stroke patients. This one involved sitting in the wheelchairs and trying to participate in exchanging objects such as large balls.

The other patients did not have a schedule with as exhausting a regimen. They might have two in the morning and two in the afternoon. Because I would be having dialysis three days a week, my schedule had to be weighted in the morning so that I had the "free time" in the afternoon to be brought on a gurney from my room on the first floor to the Hemodialysis Unit on one of the upper floors.

After lunch, which was the one meal served in the cafeteria, a transport team arrived to shuttle me up to the strangely organized Hemodialysis Unit. Dialysis is a very personal process and each dialysis technician is paired with his or her patient who requires dialysis. The first technician who was assigned to hook me up to the dialyzer was a no-nonsense pro. When I insisted that I needed the smallest gauged needles for the procedure, he mocked me. He told me it was time to grow up, that I had been babied long enough. At this point my fistula was almost five months old and that larger gauged needles would make the dialysis less painful. In spite of the direct and shaming way he delivered this message the fact that he said it would be less painful intrigued me. I consented to try the larger needles. Dialysis is a very painful and agitating procedure, yet the three hours were a little more endurable than before, but I was very glad when it was over.

When I was returned to my room, I met for the first time, the Filipina woman, who would be my primary nurse for almost all of my stay at KFRC. At first I was very apprehensive. As a Gay man I have never appeared before a woman totally naked. On the other hand I had frequented Gay nude beaches in the nude and sometimes enjoyed sexual dalliances with them in these highly eroticized locations. But women, never. When I learned that she would be responsible for bathing me, naked, in a shower-wheelchair, I was shocked and angered. This seemed to be a total violation of my civil rights.

As if this wasn't bad enough, my stay at KFRC happened during the week of July 4th, and July 4th being a national holiday, the rehab staff had the day off, and there was absolutely nothing for us to do. When I had my stroke, it had partially been triggered by the nurse in charge of my section of the Dialysis factory. That anger had never really been resolved, it had just simmered. But the frustration and anger that had been simmering over the past week and a half boiled into full rage.

The charge nurse who had oversight over all the patients in KFRC noticed my level of agitation and alerted both my social worker and the psychologist who were available to any patient who needed extra help. The psychologist had identified me as such a patient and these professionals wasted no time in hastening to my aid. The two women were helpful. They tried to address my concerns. They actually made a difference. I was still angry and frustrated about everything that had happened to me since both my diagnosis with End Stage Renal Disease which required me to have dialysis, and also since my 1993 AIDS diagnosis, but at least I returned to be willing to participate in my rehabilitation, now suspended for a day by the 4th of July.

With classes resuming the following day, things settled back into the regime that had preceded it. Meanwhile, I had many visitors including my partner and soon-to-be-spouse, Steve and our dog, Bo, my parents, my sister and her husband, many friends from both Oakland and San Francisco and other relatives. I did not realize how important these visitors were, not only for morale, but for something I had not considered.

One of our no-rehab activities over the weekend was a meeting of all male patients who had suffered a stroke. My stroke had had a significant effect on my speech. That is why one of my classes was Speech Therapy. But what was so illustrative about this discussion was that the men who had not been visited by family and friends had much more difficulty with this exercise than men, like me, who had had some or many visitors.

But the absolute favorite visit was when Steve brought Bo, our dog, to see me. He wasn't allowed inside of the facility; Steve brought Bo to the breezeway outside of the hospital adjacent to the parking lot and we had a wonderful visit, I in my wheelchair, Bo held by Steve on his leash.

The rest of my stay at KFRC was relatively uneventful, classes, dialysis, discussions with the friends I had met and the occasional hypoglycemia event due to overdosing for a meal I refused to eat. There was one horrifying event late one night in our four-man room. The guy whose bed was next to mine and was surely the most fragile patient in the room went into a code blue situation and it seemed like all hell had broken loose. Suddenly doctors, nurses and paramedics invaded the relative quiet of a hospital room. Alarms sounded and we thought our roommate had died.

The medical team was able to get my older neighbor into intensive care and to restore our room to the peace that had preceded the "Code Blue" alert. We were all relieved but equally alarmed and disturbed.

I would be remiss if I did not tell you how my relationship with my nurse evolved. At first I was very annoyed that my nurse who was going to bathe me was a Filipina woman who did not speak the best English. I have no problem appearing in front of men completely nude. I have gone to all male nude beaches frequently; after all I am a Gay man. But being naked in front of any woman is totally foreign to me.

Yet, this wonderful woman won me over. In spite of the fact that most of our meetings happened in the shower, with me in the nude and her gowned in water-proof protective gear, we got to know each other pretty well. She told me that her early nursing experience had been in Germany. She told me that in Germany nurses are called kranken-schwester – literally translated kranken means sick or for the sick and schwester, where the "w" is pronounced like an English "v" and means sister, a reminder of the pre-Reformation days when the sick were attended by religious women who addressed with title Sister, the word that is still used in England for their nurses.

Anyway, my Filipina nurse and I would start laughing hysterically every time I addressed her as "Kranken-Schwester." When it was time for me to go home, we both cried as we said our Goodbyes. My psyche and my thinking had been changed by this woman.

At the end of two weeks, my time at KFRC had come to an end. I know I was not yet fully re-habilitated, as time went on I questioned if I would ever be returned to the way my body worked before June 24, 2008. I don't know if Medicare had made the decision that I had had as much rehab as they allowed, or if it was Kaiser's decision, or if they really felt that they had done as much as they could, or if they really meant that they wanted me to be home for a week before Steve and I would stand in front of a San Francisco Justice of the Peace and recite our marriage vows. No matter, who made the decision, when July 15th dawned I had to be ready to display my ability to do the things my rehab coaches had taught me. Steve would follow me for each visit to each coach. I was given exercises to perform at home and then we packed and Steve drove me home, my first time there since my June 24th stroke.

One of the big challenges that had to be resolved before I could be released was where I was going to have my dialysis after KFRC. After much discussion, I was going to be returned to Dr. Yankulin and that my dialysis care would continue in the same unit where it had begun, in San Francisco's Kaiser Hospital, directly under Dr. Yankulin's supervision.

Chapter 20

Dialysis Returns Me

To San Francisco

First of all, I was so grateful to be leaving Vallejo and on my way to a home I had not seen in three weeks. I was assisted by my quad-cane which made walking safer. I felt that I had not been fully rehabilitated, but there was general consensus that it was time for me to go home. The consensus was uniting me, Kaiser, Medicare and the KFRC staff. Enough money had been spent on me.

Behind the scenes, the KFRC staff and Kaiser San Francisco's Hemodialysis had been struggling to find a dialysis chair in the unit where I had begun my dialysis journey some four months prior. Meanwhile, Steve had been working overtime to find family members and friends who would be willing to drive me from Oakland to dialysis in San Francisco and pick me up to bring me home. The thought of me taking public transportation was so frightening that everyone shook in horror.

Since my first full day at home was a dialysis day, my ride arrived promptly and I and my cousin and his wife had a delightful ride from my home to the hospital. It was so wonderful to see Dr. Yankulin again, and to be fully under his care again.

This time, in the San Francisco Hemodialysis Unit, I had my own special bed. Everyone else was in a chair. My special bed was in a sequestered private room. I arrived with all the apprehension I usually brought to dialysis, but everyone was so nice to me, so different from the RAI factory which had sent me into the rage precipitating my disabling stroke, that I felt much relief. From the start I developed affection for the entire Hemodialysis Unit's staff.

As I told you in the previous chapter, the staff at KFRC had made getting to our wedding on July 22nd one of my rehabilitation process goals. Steve and I went to San Francisco City Hall for the actual ceremony. Steve joked that one of the vows should be "For better 'cause it can't get any worse." I am not sure how much of a joke this was and how much he really meant it.

Then about ten days after the wedding and two weeks after my release from rehabilitation at KFRC all hell broke loose. I started to feel terrible, not just the malaise that accompanies dialysis but such terrible vomiting and diarrhea that I became quite aware that I was in grave danger. I could not eat, I could not even swallow. In my moments alone in bed I realized that I was very close to death and tried to accept that reality.

Steve got so frustrated and concerned that he called my cousin Veronica to ask her to help. Both of them were also desperately trying to contact Dr. Yankulin, but since the crisis happened on a Sunday, the odds of reaching him were quite out of favor. When Veronica walked into our bedroom, she later told me that she could smell death, I don't know what that means but she had much more experience with these kinds of things.

Steve went to the store to see if he could find anything I could eat or drink. While he was out shopping, Dr.

Yankulin called. After asking me about my condition, he asked to speak to Veronica. Not knowing that I had him on speaker, he asked Veronica if she thought I looked like I was dying. In spite of the fact that I could hear both sides of their conversation, Veronica told the truth. She said I definitely looked like I was dying. Presumptively, he diagnosed my condition as C-dif, Clostridium Difficile. Clostridium Difficile, the curse of the nursing home, is a rapidly moving bacterial infection, which without treatment can cause death in a matter of days. Dr. Yankulin immediately decided that I needed to start the drug vancomycin as soon as possible. When Steve arrived home from his search for food I might eat he was immediately sent to the pharmacy to retrieve the desperately needed medication. It was a harrowing several days, but Dr. Yankulin was right. The vancomycin worked and I recovered as well as any kidney failure patient on dialysis could recover.

Dialysis is a really obnoxious procedure. First of all there are the needles which hurt every time they are inserted. Secondly, there's the overheating of the blood in the dialyzer which of course raises one's temperature and induces a drowsy condition. Thirdly, it causes nausea depending on what has been eaten before the procedure. And finally, it is very tedious, there are three hours of ennui preceded by a half hour of pain and followed by similar pain.

There were several things that helped to make this tolerable. One was the kind and gentle way the nurses treated me. Two was Dr. Yankulin's weekly visits and encouragement.

Despite the Oakland cardiologist's dismissal of the possibility of cardiac catherization, and by implication the possibility of a lifesaving kidney transplant, Dr. Yankulin was not going to give up. He was committed to getting me a transplant, literally, no matter what. After New Year's he arranged for my cardiac catherization despite the Oakland cardiologist's nixing doubts.

It seemed that I had changed universes just by crossing the Bay Bridge once again. Unlike the Oakland team, Dr. Yankulin and his San Francisco cohorts were definitely on my side. From July until December, Steve would not allow me to travel by myself to San Francisco. I was not only dependent on friends and relatives to take me to dialysis and bring me home; I went nowhere without my quad cane.

There were other medical issues that had been put on hold during my sojourn under the supervision of Oakland Kaiser, but once I got back to San Francisco, Dr. Yankulin's staff and colleagues could not do enough for me. Appointments to remove several of the cancers Dr. Goldstein had discovered on my shoulders and shins were arranged but the biggest change was the acceleration to move me along the path to transplant.

Interestingly, the Kaiser Doctors seemed to be reluctant to share bad news with their clients and didn't reveal the severity of conditions until the medical "Rubicon" has been crossed. I think I was in a lot worse shape than I thought I was. In fact there came a day when Dr. Yankulin told me that he did not know how he was going to keep me alive.

In the meanwhile, as I said earlier, my stroke and my return to Dr. Yankulin and his much more aggressive care completely changed the trajectory to transplant. Amazingly, after initially having been shut down by the Oakland Kaiser medical staff, I was put into overdrive.

In addition to the scheduling of my cardiac catherization, there were many appointments scheduled with various arms of UCSF. Dr. Yankulin told me that I was accruing time from the moment of my first intake interview at UCSF which happened in 2007. The reason that this time is so significant is that rarely does a person who needs a kidney transplant get one until he or she has been on the waiting list for from five to seven years.

Fortunately for me there was another option. Persons on the standard waiting list are vying for kidneys from all potential kidney donors, both living and cadaver, a universe of persons with no particularly remarkable traits. The other list is called the High Risk Donor List. This list comprises Gay men (obviously HIV-), sex workers, former prisoners, and former drug addicts. Of course the persons on the High Risk Donor List had to have healthy kidneys.

This group was much smaller than the general list but also, a little scarier to most patients, hence this list portended a much shorter wait time. Dr. Yankulin had advised me that I put myself on this list rather than the larger but slower list.

So, there were a number of aggressive interviews determining whether or not I was actually an appropriate candidate to receive a donated kidney. Since I had been diagnosed with an opportunistic infection which gave me a diagnosis of what was called, in 1993, I was identified as having full-blown AIDS. Before the advent of protease inhibitors and then the so-called "AIDS cocktail," no person who was HIV+ or diagnosed with "full blown AIDS" had ever been allowed to receive a kidney transplant. Thus something that received greater scrutiny was my T-cell count, viral load and my ability to take the many drugs in my "cocktail" on a regular basis, enough to keep the indicator numbers stable. The investigators also wanted to know about the stability of my home, my ability to afford the drugs that would be used to protect the transplanted kidney, and my use or non-use of alcohol and non-prescription drugs. These interviews were exhausting and frightening. I felt like I was being investigated by the FBI.

Then there were the picayune points. I really don't remember all the things that were investigated except for a scary point which actually turned out to be a misunderstanding on my part. After my three episodes of pneumocystis pneumonia in 1993 and 1994 when the pentamidine, used to treat these consecutive illnesses, caused me to become a diabetic, I was given prednisone. At the time of my diagnosis, Dr. Hill had prescribed prednisone, which often causes a rise in blood sugar. Dr. Hill had informed me of this, but I had been too overwhelmed by the diagnosis of diabetes. Instead, I interpreted my problems with prednisone as an allergy. Since prednisone is inevitably used as one of the anti-rejection medicines used to protect the transplanted kidney from rejection, this was very troubling to the kidney gatekeepers at UCSF. Everyone on the Kaiser team was skeptical about my so-called allergy. Finally, my primary doctor, Dr. Follansbee, dug in and tracked down the reference in my medical chart from 1994. Most of the data in all Kaiser charts had been digitalized from the early 2000's, however this was not the case with artifacts from the 1990s. Dr. Follansbee found the chart and was able to read Dr. Hill's very illegible writing. The chart said what everyone else already knew: prednisone causes blood sugar spikes.

The other hurdles, by this point, had been cleared and on July 16th I was approved for a kidney transplant to be done at UCSF. I was told to be close to a telephone because a kidney could become available at any point. I continued to attend my thrice weekly dialysis appointments, but I was much more on edge. When one thinks about how long some dialysis patients have had to wait on the "normal" list to get to the point where I was, my impatience was bordering on the obnoxious. Every time the telephone rang in our house, Steve and I jumped, ran to the phone and then we were so disappointed when the caller turned out to be someone other than the UCSF transplant coordinator.

On Monday, July 27, 2009, I went to my afternoon dialysis appointment. I had a very annoying skin infection on my face which had prevented me from shaving. One of my favorite nurses had put me on the dialysis machine that day. I had talked to Dr. Yankulin when he visited the unit. I expressed my annoyance about the anxiety I was experiencing while waiting for the transplant call. We talked about my facial infection and I returned home in the way in which I had become familiar. I took the 38 Geary MUNI bus to the Temporary Transbay Terminal, boarded the P-Piedmont bus which after crossing the bridge dropped me right in front of our condo building, and prepared to spend a quiet Monday night at home.

The following day, Tuesday, July 28th was going to be a typical Tuesday. After watering my plants on our deck, Steve was going to drive me to Gold's Gym for my usual non-dialysis day workout.

Before I had gone out on the deck to water the plants, I decided to call the UCSF transplant coordinator to let her know how much anxiety I had been experiencing during the twelve days since I had been placed on the active transplant list. She tried to reassure me and offered counselling with someone who dealt with patients like me, consumed with anxiety. I thanked her, telling her I would think about that, all the time deciding in my own mind that I would never participate in something like that. Instead I resigned myself to doing what was in front of me; I went outside and started watering our plants.

In my depressed and resigned state, as I was watering the deck plants, I heard the phone ring. Since Steve was inside, he answered the call. He walked out onto the deck alerting me that the call was from UCSF. My immediate response was, "What do they want now?" He handed me the phone and with a somewhat annoyed voice I said, "Hello." The caller, having confirmed I was the person she was trying to reach, immediately told me, "We have a kidney for you." I was so amazed that I was hardly able to respond.

Once I hung up the phone I moved like a mad man. The first thing I did was tell Steve and then called my parents. When I told my mother the source of the kidney, a 27 year old man who had recently been in a catastrophic accident, having just been released from prison, her first words were, "We'll pray for him and his family."

I made sure the "Go-bag" I had been instructed to pack once I had heard that I had been placed at the top of the list of potential kidney transplant candidates was ready. Then I jumped into the shower and shaved my torso. Having been in the hospital so many times, I knew that the nurses would indiscriminately attach vital sign electrodes paying no attention to my hirsute body. The hair not only prevented the stickers from staying in place, removing them without being shaved was torture.

Having shaved showered and dressed I was ready for the ride to UCSF. Steve and I jumped in the car. We were expected by the transplant team by 1 PM. Our lives were about to change radically.

Chapter 21

Kidney Transplant at UCSF

Now you may be asking yourself why I, as a Kaiser patient, had to go to UCSF for my kidney transplant. The reason is rather complicated. As I described to you earlier, Kaiser San Francisco had had an embryonic kidney transplant program but something very unfortunate happened. At one point something went terribly wrong. I am not completely clear on what happened but what I have heard is that a potential transplant candidate had sued Kaiser and the settlement was that any Kaiser patient who required a transplant would have the operation done at UCSF by UCSF surgeons and monitored by the same team for the transplant recipient's life.

Steve and I arrived at UCSF in plenty of time. The midday Tuesday summer traffic was very light. We arrived so early that the coordinator was not even ready for us. Eventually I was admitted to UCSF's Long Hospital to the 9th Floor Kidney Unit. Steve assisted me in getting into my hospital gown and settled in my bed. Unlike Kaiser, it was a two-bed room, which seemed odd to me because of the tremendous risk of infection to which transplant patients are subject. But at that point of placement I was the only patient in the room.

Shortly after I was settled in my bed, the procession started. The first transplant team member was Laurie Carlsen, the actual transplant coordinator. She began to enumerate the various transplant team members who would be visiting me. At the top of the list was the female surgeon who would be performing the transplant operation, Dr. Fang. Along with her were the interns and associates who would be assisting her, Dr. Fang told me that the team expected the harvested kidney to arrive by 8 PM and the transplant operation would happen shortly after she had carefully verified that the kidney was an appropriate match for me. This was news to me. I thought when I got the call from UCSF to get to the hospital as quickly as possible the kidney would already be in place. I learned right then that the kidney had not yet been harvested, that the donor, who was on life support, having been rendered brain dead in an accident in Los Angeles was still in the hospital, and that the kidney would not even be harvested until I, and probably the other recipients of his vital organs, who had also been summoned to appropriate hospitals, gowned, and tested, were expectantly awaiting their life-saving operations. I thought everything would have been in place by the time I got to the hospital. It wasn't and all I would have to do was wait, watch television, try to read and try to put my impatience on hold – an almost impossible feat.

Then there was a consult with the insulin pump specialist who in turn consulted with my diabetes nurse educator, Nugget Burkhart. The two of them agreed that I would be able to continue to wear my insulin pump and maintain my basal rate and blood sugar control during the operation.

Several times, Laurie Carlsen, the transplant coordinator, came in to review the medication regime I would have to follow after transplant. She also acquainted me with the device that would allow me to dose myself with pain medication whenever I felt pain in the places where the surgery would be performed.

Then the waiting began in earnest. I kept getting updates about the time the kidney was set to arrive, and it kept getting pushed back later and later. First it was 9 PM, then 10, then shortly after midnight. The various messengers informed me that once the kidney was harvested it would be driven by limousine from the Los Angeles hospital where it would be loaded onto an airplane at LAX. Once it arrived at SFO, it would be loaded onto another limousine and driven to UCSF. Once it arrived at UCSF, Dr. Fang and her assistants would verify once again that the harvested kidney was an appropriate match for me.

But these messengers kept coming in to inform me that the kidney was still not "here." I became more and more anxious, more and more fearful and more and more impatient. But the clock kept ticking, and TV programs kept getting more and more boring. Finally, around 2:30 AM on Wednesday, July 29th 2009 I was informed that that the kidney had arrived and Dr. Fang had begun her verification. I was informed that the kidney of a 27 year old cadaver donor was a perfect match for me, every point was a match. I was told that the gurney to take me to surgery would arrive momentarily. The butterflies in my stomach went from high to astronomical.

Suddenly the gurney arrived, I placed myself on the gurney and was wheeled down the hall of the ninth floor of Long Hospital past a room guarded by two police officers; a prisoner, from I don't know where, was also getting a kidney. The transport personnel loaded me on the elevator and we proceeded to the operating floor: three in Long Hospital.

San Francisco summers are frequently colder than its winters and 2009 was no exception, particularly on Parnassus Heights, where UCSF sits. So as I waited in the breezeway outside of the Operating Room on the third floor of Long Hospital, in spite of the blankets covering me, I was trembling from nerves as well as cold. Despite the fact that I had been summoned for the operation I wondered why I had to wait yet again.

After what seemed like an interminable wait, the operating room doors opened and I was wheeled in. I was greeted by Dr. Fang and her assistants and nurses. Since I already had an IV in my arm, one of the nurses attached another bag to my IV and suddenly a mask was placed over my nose and mouth, which brought back memories of the tonsillectomy I had had in 1955 and in seconds I was out cold. The nurse had told me to start counting backwards from 10 and I think I got to 8.

The next moment of consciousness occurred somewhere around 9 AM. There was a hand very near my groin and I was totally alarmed by this feeling. As I was reviving, I asked, "What is going on?" The orderly doing whatever he was doing answered, "You're in the Recovery Room. I'm just making sure your dressing is properly in place. I'm preparing you for your return to your room."

Within minutes I was wheeled back to the elevator and returned to my 9th Floor room, which I found was no longer occupied by only me. I had a roommate, but I was in no condition to deal with him. I was exhausted, and I still had a lot of anesthetic in my body. But I was not so tired that I did not call Steve or my parents. All three were very relieved that I had survived the operation, but we had to see if the transplanted kidney was really working. In addition to a lot of anesthesia I had my self-dosing pump delivering relatively high doses of Norco, a very strong liquid narcotic to eliminate any pain I might be feeling.

Also, I was given a high dose of emotionally manipulating prednisone. As I mentioned before, prednisone does force rises in blood sugar. It also has a direct effect on the emotion centers in the brain and as noon approached I started to experience waves of sadness. Since my last dialysis had occurred on the Monday before the UCSF transplant call, as 1 PM approached it dawned on me that if I weren't at UCSF I would be entering the Kaiser Hospital Hemodialysis Unit. For the past year this had been an integral part of my week. In spite of the fact that I hated dialysis, I had become dependent on the Hospital team and actually had grown to love them. Suddenly I was cut off from them, I no longer needed them, I no longer had a reserved seat at my dialysis time. I missed them all terribly. My feelings, my loss, and the prednisone had brought these emotions to a boil. Despite that I now had a perfectly functioning transplanted kidney and was peeing regularly without difficulties, I wished that I was still in the nurturing environment of the Kaiser San Francisco Hospital Hemodialysis Unit. I missed all the nurses and particularly Dr. Yankulin. And as I had these thoughts coupled with the emotional reactions, due to the high doses of prednisone I was taking, I started to cry. These tears were not tears of joy for the amazing fact that I had now been given a much better chance of living a normal life and that dialysis was over. They were tears of sadness for being separated from a cocoon that had cared for me for the past year.

Now, one of the most important changes that the transplanted kidney did for me was restoring the ability to pee regularly. It came at the expense of very heavy narcotics to block the significant pain wrought by the surgery. At first, at the slightest twinge of pain, I pressed the drug administering button with reckless abandon, completely ignorant of the way this would disturb my other elimination process. At first, no staff, nurse or doctor made a big deal about my apparent constipation. But that was about to change.

Typically, the release date for a transplant recipient was three or four days after receipt of said transplanted kidney. But this release date was based on the restoration of regular bowel movements. And my bowels were not cooperating, they were not moving. My overuse of the IV

Narco had brought my bowel system to a standstill. Now, I imagine one of the reasons for the quick release of transplant patients is economic. It costs a lot to care for patients who are at extreme risk of infection and reaction. The other is infection. Hospitals are one of the most dangerous places for patients with lowered immune systems, and since it's necessary to trick the body into accepting a foreign organ, medications like cyclosporine and prednisone do the tricking. Hence, the UCSF staff really tried to do everything possible to send me home, but nothing worked, and I continued to suffer extreme constipation. I had stopped punching the Narco button around the second day, but that was not enough. The damage had been done.

Now, I had never been a drinker of coffee which tends to have a constipation relieving effect, but I had reached the desperation point. Although I did not drink coffee, I love coffee milkshakes, and they on occasion had had a similar constipation relieving effect. Early on the morning of my eighth day in the hospital, I begged my friend Aaron to find me a coffee milkshake somewhere in San Francisco. After some research in the area close to Parnassus Heights, he reported that none could be found. He said one thing that could be found easily was iced coffee, and being desperate I responded that something is better than nothing, and gave him the go-ahead.

Aaron arrived about a half an hour later with the magic elixir. I drank it immediately and within a half an hour I had my first bowel movement in eight days. The elixir had worked and the last hurdle preventing me from being discharged from UCSF and going home was cleared. When the doctors and nurses heard this glorious news they immediately made the necessary arrangements and prepared me for discharge.

Now, it was not just a "You can go home" statement. The discharge instructions were very complicated. Among them was the reminder that I would have weekly outpatient appointments and blood draws at the hospital for at least a couple of months.

Once we were finally out of the hospital and Steve had brought the car to the circular driveway in front of Long Hospital to meet my wheelchair, we were on our way. As I remember, it was a little before 4 PM when we drove away from UCSF headed first to the pharmacy at the Kaiser San Francisco Medical Center at 2238 Geary Boulevard. And, as usual, there was a very long line and wait. When we got to the head of the line, every single drug I had been taking plus the new anti-rejection medicines to protect my newly received transplanted kidney were in a bag, and there were a lot. The bag was very heavy.

Despite the fact that we were in the month of August, which is usually a time of many vacations of San Francisco Bay Area workers, the traffic heading to the bridge was rush-hour intense. We knew it was going to be a slog.

We finally got home, and since I hadn't seen our dog Bo since the day I went to UCSF for the transplant, Steve was concerned about how crazy Bo would be when he finally saw me. He went into the condo to hold Bo so that he wouldn't knock me over with his enthusiasm. But something unexpected happened. Instead of breaking the restraints Steve had placed on him, he looked at me with that curious head movement, what we humans would call a quizzical gaze. He was confused. He didn't bark, he recognized my face and body, but, since dogs have sense of smell 100,000 stronger than us humans, I did not smell like the Frank that had bid him goodbye as I left for UCSF. If I wanted proof of how much my transplanted kidney had changed me, Bo gave me a true answer, the old urea ridden blood was now being continually cleansed. I smelled different and that was an amazing change for me but one causing total confusion for Bo.

As soon as Steve fed Bo, instead of preparing dinner, he joined me at the dining room table to sort and count my medications, new and old, and place the whole new set in my pill tray. Because of the numerous new medications and the changes in dosing of old ones, this took a long time.

Finally, after filling the tray, we had dinner, the first in our home that I had enjoyed since starting dialysis, 16 months prior to my return home.

I forgot to tell you about another inconvenience that resulted from my transplant operation. The kidney was definitely working. It was delivering urine to my bladder on a very regular basis. But in order to protect the kidney that had been sewn to my bladder, a very inconvenient and uncomfortable catheter had been inserted in my penis and attached to a Foley bag, which had to be emptied regularly. This would not be removed until my first post-transplant clinic appointment.

The removal of the catheter was both painful and embarrassing especially having a woman have to remove it from my very tired penis. I don't like having women see my penis and this made the whole appointment that much more uncomfortable.

Prior to the appointment with Laurie and the Nurse Practitioner, who would remove my catheter, I had the first of many weekly blood draws, and these blood draws were monumental in size. I think the phlebotomist drew around fifteen tubes of blood. It was amazing, and it would be happening every week for the next several months. The good news is that the medical team was very pleased with the first blood draw and appointment.

Steve and I went home grateful that the first week at home had gone so well. One of the special precautions we had to make to make sure I was not infected by unwanted contact with suspicious infections was to confine me to our home and to require any visitor to sanitize his or her hands before entering the condo, and anyone with a respiratory infection was banned from visiting. Also, during the first month I was not allowed to ride public transportation, attend Mass or go to 12 step meetings and no one could get close enough to hug or kiss me.

The first month was very boring. We did, however, drive to Santa Rosa to see my parents. After we returned home, while I was doing my pill tray fill on Friday evening I became tremendously hot, in fact I was sweating. Now, September and October in the Bay Area are typically the hottest months of the year, so I wasn't particularly surprised that I was feeling the heat or being more than usually warm. Still, I thought I better check my temperature. When I took my temperature I was shocked that my temperature had breached 100^0. For a person whose temperature is rarely above 97^0, this was shocking. It was after hours on a Friday night, so I called the Kidney Transplant Emergency line at UCSF. The operator connected me to the Transplant Doctor on call, and he told me to come in to the Emergency Room immediately. Just as he had done on the occasion of my kidney transplant, and every other emergency, Steve drove me back across the Bay Bridge, and across the city. I was triaged with amazing swiftness and almost instantly placed in an Emergency bay for immediate examination. All the anomalous conditions were observed and I was quickly transferred back to the 9th Floor, the Kidney Transplant Floor of Long Hospital, the place where this new journey had begun.

Nevertheless, somehow in the month or so after my transplant operation, my weakened immune system had left me open to infection. Basically, the UCSF kidney team was able to tweak my medications and give me the necessary tune-up to get me back on my feet, and by the time the weekend was over, I was ready to return home. Steve and I were so relieved, we returned home with renewed hope, UCSF was able to handle this first crisis.

I was still not able to return to public life, go to the gym, go to church, or travel by myself, that was still months away. But during this time I was succumbing to cabin fever. And then just about a month after my first crisis, it happened again.   The first crisis was in late September, the next crisis happened in October, and the same drill was followed.

By November my condition had become more stable. We hosted Thanksgiving for my family. At the time I did not know that it would be the last one I would share with my father. 2009 was the ninetieth anniversary of his birth and on December the 6th we celebrated with a big party for him and his family, his siblings and their families. It was the first time I had seen many of my relatives since my transplant.

By this time the frequency of blood tests and UCSF kidney visits had diminished. Steve was still taking me to the UCSF appointments and the Kaiser appointments but I was straining at the leash. I wanted freedom again.

When an appointment with Dr. Goldstein came in early December, Steve, against his better judgment, allowed me to travel by myself to and from Kaiser French to see Dr. Goldstein. Since Christmas was approaching, I decided to go to Macy's to try to get a box for a present for Steve. I had called Steve from Kaiser French before boarding the 38-Geary bus. I hadn't told him of my Macy's detour. Unfortunately, while I was in Macy's I began to feel dizzy. Something was wrong. I decided, as I descended the escalators, that I had better get some sugar. I went to Walgreen's on my way to the Powell Street BART station. But instead of consuming the sugar immediately, I rushed to the station and got on board the first train. I could have eaten the candy upon sitting, but instead of eating it, I immediately passed out. Since the BART train was underground in San Francisco and then in the Transbay tube, I was in relative darkness. It was easy to remain somewhat comatose in my hypoglycemic state. My blood sugar had fallen well below the safe level.

As we emerged into open areas, including the departure from the Transbay Tube, I was thrust into the light, but in my dangerous hypoglycemic state I felt like I was back in Europe travelling on a fast train. I didn't call Steve from West Oakland as I usually had in the past. After the short time in light the train and I were plunged again into relative darkness, and I returned to my half-conscious state every time the train returned above ground.

Since Steve had been expecting me to call him from the West Oakland BART Station so he could pick me up at 20th and Broadway, he began frantically trying to call me after

12:30 PM. And in his panic, he called BART police to alert them about my possible medical emergency on the train which resulted in absolutely no response. About 1 PM, when the Pittsburg/Bay Point Train arrived at the Martinez Station I heard my cell phone ring for the first time since boarding the train. An angry Steve told me to get off the train and eat the candy I had purchased in San Francisco. He told me to take the next San Francisco bound train and that he would meet me at MacArthur Station. He was very angry at me for my screw-up and at himself for permitting me to take my first solo trip to San Francisco.

Once we got home, we decompressed and had lunch. We called my cousin, Veronica, whom Steve had contacted in the panic that ensued when he was unable to find me.

Anyway, it was December and we were preoccupied with our preparation for Christmas. Steve resumed taking me to my many appointments including my UCSF appointments. At one of these, he decided to seek a new job as a Senior Executive Assistant at UCSF. In fact, the recruiter was so impressed with Steve's resume and skills that he arranged an interview for Steve with the manager who supervised such employees and she forwarded his application to the head of the Emergency Department where I had been treated for my two post-transplant crises in September and October. Steve got the job and his prohibition on my solo trips to San Francisco for my medical appointments came to an end. I was once again necessitated to make my journeys by myself.

For several months there were no alarming events. Then in early March my kidney numbers appeared to be going south. The words "borderline rejection" began to be bandied about. The borderline rejection immediately necessitated a kidney biopsy.

The biopsy happened in mid-March 2010. Steve was already working at UCSF, and he had driven to work that day so that he would be able to take me home. I did arrive for the biopsy on my own steam. And yet I was terrified. The idea of a doctor sticking a large hypodermic needle in my lower abdomen to withdraw a portion of my recently inserted kidney to determine if there had actually been a borderline rejection was nothing short of abhorrent. Still I knew I had to endure this assault in order to definitively find out if the borderline rejection was indeed true.

Waiting for the biopsy was daunting; somewhat like the wait I had had for the transplant operation. When it happened it was quite unpleasant. A Muslim female doctor wearing a head scarf was the physician performing the biopsy. Those scarves bother me anyway, and being essentially naked in front of any woman is something I do not like. As she pushed the hypodermic needle into my abdomen and then kidney it was very uncomfortable, but it was very quick and then it was over. I was so relieved. I was wheeled back to the dressing area, got dressed and waited for Steve and then we went home.

As in most of my diverse medical problems, I actually was the cause of the borderline rejection my kidney had experienced. After my transplant operation, three drugs were in my anti-rejection regime. The three were prednisone, myfortic, and cyclosporine. The cyclosporine was the drug most subject to degradation due to exposure. The cyclosporine capsules come in a vacuum sealed packet, which must be opened just prior to consumption. The packets are very difficult to open, they are so well-sealed. So to make the consumption easier, I unsealed a whole bunch of capsules and put them in a much less tightly sealed pill container. At first no one noticed any difficulty. Several times a month, I was required to have blood drawn to determine if the trough level was high enough to protect my new kidney. But starting in February it was clear that something was going wrong. My cyclosporine had been falling below the protective level and other blood tests had less than optimal readings, hence the demand for the biopsy.

Sometimes, events in this story overlap themselves and what follows is a case of such overlap. The accident that broke my hand will be the subject of the next chapter, but it precedes the event that follows.

When the biopsy was reviewed it was determined that yes, there had been a borderline rejection and drastic measures were deemed necessary. A taper dose of prednisone was immediately ordered. And I started it at the very high dose of 60 mg. As I noted in the discussion of the immediate effect of the post-transplant medications, high doses of prednisone cause almost uncontrollable spikes in blood sugar and wild emotional swings of troubling proportions.

My next UCSF appointment was with the Italian physician Dr. Valenti. At my appointment with Dr. Valenti, he told me to continue the course of prednisone and said he felt that as this was a borderline rejection it more than likely would be repairable and by the time I finished the three week course of prednisone the kidney should be back to normal. I didn't tell him or Laurie Carlsen about my mistake with the cyclosporine capsules, but I immediately returned to taking cyclosporine directly from the vacuum sealed packaging in which they came rather than unsealing the capsules months before the dosages.

After this appointment the maintenance of my kidney began to have a relatively uncomplicated path. But at this point I must discuss the automobile accident that had just happened the week after I started the high taper dose of prednisone.

Chapter 22

Auto Accident

My friend David and I are big fans of Alfred Hitchcock's classic San Francisco based movie, *Vertigo*. We liked the movie so much that we decided to visit the San Francisco locations used in the movie in the order in which they occurred in the film. David had Monday's off from his job with the State of California, so we scheduled the visit for the second Monday of April 2010.

We had been to a meeting together the night before our scheduled trip to San Francisco. I was going to buy a tank of gas for David's car so that we would not waste time on Monday morning getting gas and could immediately drive to San Francisco. We had been to a meeting at the west side of Lake Merritt on Lakeshore Avenue. As we left the meeting we had to proceed through the underpass under I-580. The gas station was just beyond the underpass. As we cruised toward the stoplight that controls the traffic under I-580, it appeared to David that we would be able to make it through the intersection before the light turned red. The far left lane in the opposite direction is dedicated to drivers turning left to enter the eastbound onramp to I-580.

As we were entering the intersection, a pick-up truck driver gunned his engine anticipating his steep drive up the incline on-ramp and rammed his much larger vehicle into the driver's side of David's much smaller car and we were halted in our tracks.

Because of the right-side weakness caused by my stroke of June 2008, some twenty-two months prior to the accident, my almost useless right hand flew into the dashboard of David's car. The impact was so sharp that my hand hurt like hell. At that point I had no idea what damage had been done, but I knew it was bad.

By an amazing stroke of luck David escaped unscathed. Had he been less than a second faster, he probably would have been killed, or at least seriously maimed. The impact of the truck on his car had totaled it. Even so, he was able to get out of his car and come around to my side of the car. He opened the door and tried to take my hand, but it hurt so much that I screamed for him to not touch it. Instead I told him to immediately call my spouse, Steve, at home, and tell him to get to the scene of the accident.

Meanwhile, someone had dialed 911 and almost immediately a police man was approaching me. I think his car had just happened to be on the scene. Upon his approach the fire truck arrived and shortly after the fire truck, an ambulance appeared. I was quite hysterical and not exactly thinking clearly. Besides, I was still on a very high dose of prednisone due to my borderline kidney rejection, so like most persons on high doses of prednisone, I was much more emotional than I would have been had I not been on such a high dose. But it's probable that the extra prednisone made my pain less acute than it would have been had I not been on the extra prednisone.

Despite or because of the extra prednisone I was very anxious and very angry, and if the truth be told very uncooperative. The Emergency crew was excellent. They did everything possible to make me comfortable and expeditiously load me into the ambulance and drive me to Kaiser, just one exit to the west of where the accident had happened.

I was triaged very quickly at Kaiser Oakland and attended by rather unfriendly nurses and personnel in the Emergency Room. Steve arrived minutes after the ambulance had delivered me. Then the fireworks started. I had been wearing my favorite gold ring inset with a green stone and since it was on my damaged hand, it had to be removed before the inevitable swelling started. My hand was in a great deal of pain and any touching I found intolerable. The technicians ignored my pain and my protests and proceeded to use a metal saw to remove my ring. I was angry, I was scared and my pain was increasing by the minute, and my favorite ring was being destroyed. But once it was removed I was sent to the X-ray room.

For a Sunday night, I guess it was not that surprising that the Emergency Room was relatively quiet. It took very little time for me to be ushered into the actual room. While I was being prepared for the X-ray, I had a very interesting discussion with the Chinese-American X-ray tech. We discussed the Chinese Zodiac and how in the twelve signs of that zodiac every person has an unlucky year and 2010, the "Year of the Tiger," was my unlucky year. The tech told me that he knew less about the Chinese zodiac calendar than I did, but his mother always warned him when he was in his unlucky year.

Anyway, the X-rays showed that my fingers had indeed been broken in three places. My hand had to be wrapped to protect it until I could be seen in San Francisco Kaiser's Injury Clinic, which would require me to make an appointment before I could be seen and have my hand and fingers reset.

So, having been X-rayed, evaluated, suffered the severing of my favorite ring, had my hand bandaged and put in a sling, I was discharged to go home. Since it was now past 1 AM and Steve had to get home, he had left me to find a cab to bring me home.

So when I went out to the cab stand steaming mad about everything, I got into the first cab waiting but once I was seated I realized that my injured bandaged hand would be unable to close the door and told the driver that I could not close the door because of my injury. Instead of being of service, he lazily sat in his cab and infuriated me even more. When I realized that nothing was going to be done to help me, I, angered even more, exited the cab, slammed the door shot, and went back into the Oakland Emergency Room waiting area. Receiving no assistance, in spite my exhaustion, in spite of my injury, in spite of the fact that no matter how good the neighborhood, it is not wise to walk by oneself through the streets of Oakland as the time is approaching 2 AM, I decided that I would walk home storming through the streets, and thieves and menacing denizens of the night be damned. I was so angry I was ready to face any marauder. Fortunately, there were none and I made it up the steep Monte Vista hill and arrived at home around 2 AM. Steve was asleep and Bo was waiting for me near the door. I was so glad to see him that he helped me to become a little bit saner and calmer.

Monday I would have to face all the issues around insurance liability and the settlement I might receive for enduring and surviving the accident.

But the most disappointing fact of all was something that would only become clear in hindsight. The day before the accident, April 10th, I had decided that I had recovered enough from the stroke of 22 months prior that I could try to ride my bicycle. I had not ridden my new bike since several months before my June 24th, 2008 stroke and I was itching to try it. Steve only allowed me to ride around the garage but it was so wonderful to be riding a bike again. I have always found it to be the closest thing to flying without being in the air above the ground. The other thing that had happened is that I had begun playing the piano with both hands while I was still on dialysis. I had no idea how the broken fingers in my right hand would heal but my suspicion was that my recovery would not be easy.

I was so tired that it was very difficult to get ready to go to bed. I had to figure out how to remove my clothes facing the obstacle of the cast on my hand. Somehow I did, and for the first time in a longtime I had little trouble getting to sleep.

Steve had to get up early to get to work, I did not. But I had a very taxing day ahead of me. I was in pain. What little strength I had regained on my right side was lost due to the pain resulting from the three fingers being broken. I had two principal tasks for the day. The first was to make an appointment with the injury clinic in San Francisco. The other was to contact David's, the driver of the car in which I was injured, insurance carrier.

The call to Kaiser was easy; all I had to do is get my friend Lon to take me to the appointment. I certainly was unable to take public transportation, so Lon's offer to take me was a godsend. Since Steve had to work and could not take me, I was extremely grateful for Lon's offer of support.

The other call to David's car insurance carrier was more challenging. The first obstacle presented to me was that both David *and* the driver of the truck who hit us were insured by the same carrier, USAA. USAA is an insurance company specifically founded to cover American military veterans and their dependents. Both David and the other driver were such dependents. I, on the other hand, was a third party claimant with no auto insurance at all. In most accidents, where each driver is represented by a separate insurance carrier, the two of them fight it out with each other. Had they been separate carriers it might have been simpler. In the event it was very bad for me. The whole thing was further complicated by the fact that, although I was a Kaiser patient, the monetary responsibility lay with

Medicare, and they had their own complicated bureaucracy. Not only was I in shock from the trauma of the accident, I was now dazed by the complexity of the insurance morass ahead of me. I saw it was going to be an uphill climb; though I had no idea how steep it would be.

I had been advised by everyone not to settle anything but simply to open a claim. USAA told me to keep track of all the receipts I had received and would get for my expenses due to the accident. This seemed very simple. I had no idea how challenging it would become.

Following the terrible experience after my loss of the lawsuit against the DeSoto Cab Company I was particularly leery about going anywhere near a courtroom to resolve a dispute against someone who had injured me. Still, what had happened in the April 2010 car accident was completely different from what had happened on February 14, 1998. In the former incident I had found myself in a verbal dispute with the driver before he physically injured me. In the April 11, 2010 accident I was simply an injured passenger who had done nothing to cause the accident.

When I called David's insurance company I was hoping they would simply seek to find a settlement with me that would be acceptable to me and equitable. My hand had been broken, my ring had been cut, my stroke recovery had been interrupted and my sense of safety had been completely shaken. How they would repair these problems, I had no idea.

I did everything I was supposed to do. I went to San Francisco to have my hand reset so that it would heal affording me the use of my fingers. I kept track of all the expenses and had dutifully sent these to the claims department at USAA. And I decided to seek the advice of Kaiser's Member Services. To my great surprise I was informed by Member Services in May that in order to recover the losses I had incurred in the accident and the subsequent medical attention and physical therapy I would require, I would need to open up something called a "Third Party Lawsuit."

That lawsuit terrified me. I did not want to get involved with courts and lawyers again. I had been burned the first time and I had no desire to re-enter that fire. But it seemed to me that I really had no choice.

At this point, I decided to turn to my closest acquaintance who was an attorney, my brother Anthony. I had no desire to select him as my attorney, I just wanted his advice. He surprised me by telling me that he would happy to represent me as my attorney. I heaved a huge sigh of relief. It was no longer necessary to find my way through this morass by myself. I had an attorney whom I trusted and who would not try to make money on my misfortune.

The decision to open a Third Party Lawsuit and to seek my brother's advice had completely changed the course of this part of my health care journey. I had no idea what was going to happen I just wanted the lawsuit settled without entering a courtroom. I had no idea what a challenging journey it would be.

The first leg of this journey began with my brother writing a letter to USAA telling the adjusters handling my suit that he would be handling my legal affairs going forward. In May of 2010 it seemed that this would be a simple straightforward process. Yet since both drivers were covered by USAA the complications appeared very quickly. Whether David or the other driver were ultimately responsible is essentially moot, the only thing that was very clear is that the driver of the truck had broadsided David's car just missing severely damaging or killing him by inches. Just by the impact it seemed that the truck driver was responsible but if David had entered the intersection after the light had changed then he might be blamed for being in the wrong place at the wrong time. And this was the nub of the argument.

The battle had begun. And the waiting game was just as arduous. Meanwhile, I continued to receive physical therapy for my injured hand. I had been making progress on my stroke rehabilitation, which had been severely interrupted by the breaks in my hand wrought by the accident. Though I did not know this, I began to see that my stroke condition before the accident would be an obstacle to reaching a settlement.

I became more and more anxious as I watched the dilatoriness with which the insurance company was proceeding toward resolution. In addition to the slow-walking process, Kaiser, who had all the medical information, was being less than cooperative in terms of supplying all of the records germane to my treatment. My attorney was having a very difficult time securing all the available records.

The whole mess surrounding this case had become the bane of my existence. I wanted so desperately for this case to be settled, but it seemed to be a Sisyphean effort. I could get no information from anyone.

Meanwhile, something amazing happened. During the summer of 2010 Steve and I vacationed at the family cabin in Plumas County in the Feather River Canyon. Our dog, Bo, loved swimming in this small narrow river and I decided to join him in the river. Now, since the accident, I had gingerly favored my right hand. But as most folks know, swimming is a very balanced exercise, and as I swam with Bo I had to use my right hand and side. The swimming which required me to use both hands and arms for the first time since the car accident and in some ways since my stroke two years prior was a tremendous awakening.

The next morning, as Steve and I were taking Bo for his first walk of the day, I was amazed at the feelings and nerve responses which had returned to my unused hand and arm. I realized that I had discovered a previously untried path to recovery. I immediately made a decision to start swimming regularly.

But the burden of my injury and the lawsuit that accompanied it were still not moving fast enough for my sense of being wronged. I had hoped that acquiring my brother as my attorney would make things run more smoothly. Unfortunately, the opposite was true. In the fall of 2010 his arrival on the scene changed the way the insurance company behaved. They basically moved into stonewall-mode. In addition, the opening of the Third Party Lawsuit and the acquisition of an attorney made the other side become much more adversarial. It felt like the burden I had undertaken had increased exponentially.

While all these daunting circumstances surrounding the broken hand and the trauma it caused were traumatizing me, other medical things were happening. I will discuss them in the next chapter, but they must be acknowledged as I proceed in discussing the slow progress of my lawsuit.

Eventually my brother had to file a formal lawsuit due to USAA's intransigence. I wonder how this case would have been handled if the drivers had been represented by separate insurance carriers. We will never know, they were both represented by the same firm, but each would have his own lawyer, which made the case so much more complicated. Not only did they countersue me, they countersued each other. About six months after the filing of my lawsuit they asked for a deposition. Anthony never deposed the two involved in the actual accident. Their responsibility had been determined by the police.

In addition, Kaiser was being less than cooperative in providing documentation of the cost of the care they provided to me and USAA would not provide us with the policy limits of each driver's insurance. So we were more or less navigating in the dark.

Basically, USAA tried to blame all my injuries on the stroke I had had approximately two years prior to the accident, but I had experienced a great deal of recovery of my right hand function after the stroke and before the accident. In fact the day before the accident, as I said before, I had convinced Steve to allow me to ride my bicycle for the first time since my stroke. And I did, but the accident causing broken fingers and loss of function in my right hand negated any progress I had been making in playing the piano and other more subtle activities.

Following the deposition the lawyers, representing the drivers in the accident appointed by USAA, demanded an independent medical examination. I was very nervous about this, thinking this was one more attempt to discredit my claims of injury caused by the accident; but surprisingly the independent medical examination report was completely in my favor. The independent doctor determined that the accident had caused diminished right hand function and the breaking of several fingers. I was not making it up. There were X-rays taken prior to the accident and after the accident which demonstrated what the accident had caused.

Still, the old lawyerly tactic of delay and delay was used on me. Every time a settlement conference date was proposed some excuse to postpone it happened.

Finally a date was set for April of 2013. It was, by that point, three years after the April 11, 2010 accident date. We had chosen mediation so a retired lawyer mediator was in the room when we arrived in the same room where my deposition had been taken. Then the USAA lawyers claimed they still needed time to prepare. My brother went ballistic and told these unprepared lawyers he would have them sanctioned for bad faith.

Once Anthony threatened to bring sanctions for their delaying tactics, everything changed. Suddenly they were motivated to telephone directly to USAA headquarters to find out what kind of settlement they could offer. My brother asked me what kind of settlement I would accept. I gave him the number I would accept and expected that number to be augmented by the amount Kaiser and Medicare expected in reimbursement. But these reimbursement costs were still not available and we had to strike while the iron was hot.. .

In the space of five minutes, we had given our settlement number, received approval, signed a settlement agreement and were on our way home.

Before Anthony drove me back to Oakland, we made a stop at Kaiser Hospital. Our 91 year old aunt had just had knee surgery and we took the opportunity to visit her, then, jubilantly we returned to Oakland. It was such a relief to have this three year burden resolved. But it wasn't over.

As soon as the legal portion of the case resolved, suddenly, Kaiser and Medicare discovered the details of the services and expenses my accident had cost. Both wasted no time in telling me and Anthony how much of the settlement money they wanted. These costs which had not been available at any time before our mediation procedure were now available. But it was too late. These expenses that I had wanted included in the settlement were now totally excluded by my signing the settlement agreement. Fortunately my brother was able to halve the amount Kaiser and Medicare wanted, but it still was a sore point for me.

Nevertheless, the mental pain of the April 11, 2010 accident was over, the damage to my hand and fingers was permanent. I would have several stints of hand therapy but they were very non-productive. Medicare determined that enough money had been spent on me and they would not allow any more. Since I had the use of my left hand and could write with it, I would have to live the rest of my life with only one fully functioning hand.

Now it's time to switch to a completely different topic. During the time I had been occupied with my accident and lawsuit I had many other medical issues that required my attention.

Chapter 23

Skin Cancer Resurfaces

One of the unexpected consequences of a kidney transplant is the massive interference it causes in the body's most important organ of protection, the skin.

Implanting someone else's kidney in a body, no matter how close the match is, requires a battery of medications to trick a body into accepting a totally foreign organ. In my case, the drugs selected to perform this alchemy were cyclosporine, myfortic, and prednisone.

These drugs are designed to suppress the immune system which would ordinarily cause a body to reject someone else's organ. But this immune suppression decreased the ability of the immune system to accomplish this. Now, we also have to remember that unlike most transplant recipients, my body had been contending with Acquired Immune Deficiency Syndrome. Before the advent of the protease inhibitors, which changed the trajectory of virtually all persons infected with the virus, a diagnosis of AIDS was a death sentence. For persons like me who had had too much unprotected sun exposure, skin cancer was also very common. But introducing immune suppressing drugs to trick a body into accepting someone else's organ could open the path to increasing susceptibility to multiple skin cancers.

After my kidney transplant I was still having regular appointments with my dermatologist, Dr. Goldstein, at regular three month intervals. At my first appointment after transplant, Dr. Goldstein informed me, right off the bat that the frequency of my appointments would go from once every three months to every month. He had had other transplant patients who required monthly appointments. Considering my history of skin cancer prior to transplant he knew that I was at particular risk for many skin cancers.

He was so right. I had had numerous cancers removed from my forehead, shoulder, face, arms, and, the very worst, from my shin. Since skin on the shin has virtually no fat below it, cancers on shins cannot be simply excised and closed by pulling loose skin together, these wounds require grafted skin being used to replace the removed cancerous skin. In an ordinary patient a month would be necessary for a complete recovery, for me it took two months.

Back in 2001 I had had two major skin cancer surgeries on my scalp. I have described them earlier. They were performed by now retired surgeon Dr. Ward. In the weeks before starting dialysis I had had several surgeries by Dr. Simonds. There were so many occasions on which he performed surgery on me we had become good friends. When the biopsies revealed cancers on my face, other surgeons did the work, but Dr. Simonds became my most consistent skin cancer surgeon.

It wasn't as though I hadn't had difficulties with skin cancer before my transplant. Actually, a skin cancer was one of the things that convinced me that I had to start dialysis. When I was sent to a surgeon to find out if he would remove one of these cancers, he told me that he couldn't until I had had my blood cleaned by dialysis, otherwise he couldn't guarantee my ability to heal after the surgery. This convinced me it was time to start dialysis.

About two months after starting dialysis I had a major stroke which ultimately resulted in my return to Dr. Yankulin's care and having my dialysis under his supervision in the hospital in San Francisco. He was also able to more closely observe my other medical problems; including determining when it would be safe for me to have the much needed skin cancer surgery.

This surgery was not the only one. I kept having skin cancers crop up as they had been doing since 2001.

My medical situation during dialysis was indeed fragile. Dr. Yankulin remained upbeat when talking to me. However, he was very nervous. He didn't say these words to me until after my kidney transplant, but once the transplant was beyond the rejection stage he said to me, "I didn't think I could keep you alive much longer." These were extremely frightening words. I was very grateful that he had not told me this before the transplant.

After the transplant I was placed on a course of anti-rejection medicines to protect my newly received kidney. The medicines, as I mentioned before were cyclosporine, myfortic and prednisone. All of these medicines are challenging to most patients, but even more caustic to me. The one medicine that was hardest on me was myfortic.

This medicine had the unfortunate side effect of increasing my proclivity for skin cancer.

If the skin cancer issue was annoying before the transplant it became a nightmare with the addition of myfortic. My twenty year dermatologist retired in 2013 after fighting an uphill battle to catch skin cancers before they required large surgeries. He succeeded most of the time, but not every time. But he was seeing me in his office once a month. After his retirement, I had to beg his replacement to see me more frequently than his typical patients. Still on myfortic, I turned into a cancer production system.

With the three month interval between appointments it was not unusual for several new cancer lesions to be found at each appointment, and the subsequent surgeries not only inconvenienced me, they interrupted my swimming routine.

Finally, in May and June of 2015, Dr. Zipperstein, my new dermatologist, discovered seven skin cancers, including a large lesion on my scalp. The lesion on my scalp was so large that Dr. Simonds had so much difficulty closing it that the surgery was interrupted by the arrival of paramedics.

What had happened was that my problems with esophageal reflux had been exacerbated by the position in which I had been placed. As the pain increased and my depression took over I started to focus on the extremity of my condition. I began to think that what was happening to me would continue to happen to me for the rest of my life and this depressed me so much that I was in the extremity of despair. The doctor and the nurse performing this extraordinarily painful procedure heard me sobbing and asked me if I was doing OK. When I answered in the negative they immediately summoned paramedics.

The procedure was interrupted. The paramedics arrived. They wanted to take me to the Emergency Room. I refused. I knew what was wrong. And against medical advice I refused to go to the Emergency Room. Steve and I had plans for the evening. We were going to dinner and the symphony and I was not going to miss these events because I was being held against my will by the very slow Emergency Room staff.

The upshot of this catastrophe was that Dr. Simonds told me that at the next procedure he did on me it would be performed in an operating room and I would be under anesthesia.

Meanwhile as I proceeded to the next four skin cancer removal surgeries I had another endoscopy and a conference with my gastroenterologist and then my UCSF transplant doctor decided that I would no longer be required to take aspirin which was causing some of my esophageal problems and the myfortic, which was one of the principal causes of the skin cancers, could be discontinued.

No sooner had these decisions been made than I saw remarkable changes, suddenly I had a perfect skin cancer checkup for the very first time in a very long time. What a relief. I felt the decisions to remove the drugs were the right ones.

In addition to the cancer lesions that had popped up on various places on my body from my shins to my forehead and face, many actinic keratoses had been plaguing my scalp before my kidneys failed, before I started getting dialysis, and before my kidney transplant accompanied with immune suppressive drugs.   In fact I had been complaining about the continual itching all over my scalp almost from my diagnosis with AIDS. The itching scalp always reminded me of the way my whole body felt when I had Hepatitis B back in 1978. At that time it had been explained to me that this itching was caused by the fact that the liver could no longer filter the bilirubin which is what makes feces brown rather than white and that this unfiltered thick bilirubin gets stuck in the capillaries causing the insufferable itch. The itch I had been feeling since I became a diabetic reminded me of the bilirubin itch. Dr. Goldstein had tried everything, including sending me to skin experts at UCSF. These trips to UCSF had been just as useless as most of what Dr. Goldstein tried to do. So finally in 2007, well before my kidneys failed and I started dialysis on the road to transplant, Dr. Goldstein had started other patients on a new therapy which involved shining a blue light on my scalp, after my scalp had been painted with a special solution, which made my scalp skin more reactive to the intense blue light. The nurse, Raj, who administered this therapy was an old acquaintance from my CMV retinitis battle when she was assisting my ophthalmologist, Dr. Wolitz. It was great to see her again, but after the hour during which the special solution had saturated my scalp, I lasted no more than five seconds under the heat of the blue light. It felt like someone had taken an overheated griddle from the gas flames and placed it on my scalp. After jumping out of the therapeutic chair I swore that I would NEVER allow that therapy to be performed on me again.

Dr. Goldstein and Raj shook their heads and decided to look for other remedies. Then, as my kidney problems changed to End Stage Renal Disease, it seemed to everyone that I was on my road to an early death and there was no point in pursuing these scalp remedies.

Then another miracle happened, I advanced to the top of the kidney transplant list. As I told you in an earlier chapter, one of the reasons that I had advanced to the first position on the kidney transplant list is that I had chosen to be among those receiving kidneys from high risk donors. As you already know, the kidney transplant operation was a huge success. My life changed phenomenonally. And this had an effect on Dr. Goldstein. The very thin skin on my scalp which had received untold sun exposure and untold sunburns might be ready for another treatment by Raj and her blue light. Dr. Goldstein thought it was worth a try. He begged me try it again. Of course, I was just as apprehensive, as I had been after the "frying pain" debacle. But I thought, "Well, I might as well give it another try. I can always flee like I did in 2007." The good news is that something had changed; the nerves in my scalp were less sensitive than they had been before my kidney transplant.

Amazingly I survived the sixteen minute blue light exposure. And, once the burned skin flaked off, my scalp was transformed, it was virtually actinic keratosis free. Therefore, I was willing to continue with regular treatments and have continued with this to the present day.

Chapter 24

The Other End

Of the Digestive System

This chapter may be more challenging than the others. I certainly won't be offended if you skip it. But if you can handle it, as noted in the chapter title, it deals with problems that occur at the end of the digestive system, farthest from the mouth, which is the beginning of the digestive system.

When I was teaching high school, my horrible eating habits had resulted in very painful, sometimes bloody hemorrhoids. The doctor who had cared for my family for a number of years actually did what I consider butchery to my hemorrhoids. I left his office in what I considered worse shape than I had entered it. By the way, this UCSF graduate had received the prestigious gold cane, a mark of an exceptional graduate. I questioned the wisdom of according him this honor. I never saw him again.

I continued to have problems with hemorrhoids as my dalliances in Gay sex progressed. I had many visits to the Venereal Disease Clinic in Fourth Street in San Francisco. Eventually, when I received my AIDS diagnosis my problems with my anus, particularly hemorrhoids became worse.

Shortly after my diagnosis, I was referred to Dr. Stricker at Kaiser; he had to perform surgery on a hemorrhoid problem that had morphed into an anal fistula. I think anal problems are among the most difficult to repair because it is one of the areas of the body which is in constant use, no matter how troubled the anus is.

Over the years, prior to my kidney transplant, I had numerous encounters with Dr. Stricker as my anal problems persisted. I was on a number of anti-retroviral medicines which caused aggravated diarrhea if they were taken with dairy products. It took me years to discover these side effects. Once I did, I changed my eating habits and the problem was easier to handle. But once again the diarrhea problem had exacerbated the hemorrhoids and so I was always needing Dr. Stricker's expert scalpel.

Now, I had been infected with the HPV virus, the same one that can cause cervical cancer in women. Anyone who has been sexually active is more than likely exposed to this virus. One of the consequences frequently is anal warts. But when you add the problem of a lowered immune system caused by the AIDS virus, the opportunities for more anal problems are significantly increased.

Before the kidney transplant I had been followed by Dr. Stricker prophylactically and potential outbreaks were addressed as they happened. But after the kidney transplant and the addition of immune suppressive drugs accompanying it, just as my skin cancer issues had ballooned, so had the new problem of anal dysplasia increased.

By this time a new doctor had been brought to Kaiser's HIV care team, Dr. Joe Long. Part of his new practice was dedicated to the care of those of us AIDS patients who had a pre-disposition to more aggressive anal dysplasia.

My first visit with Dr. Long went very badly. He tried to treat every single instance of anal dysplasia and I left so traumatized that I had to make an appointment with Dr. Stricker to repair the damage Dr. Long had done. But the next time I saw Dr. Long he was much gentler.

It was several years before I was able to convince my UCSF transplant doctor to remove the most pernicious anti-rejection medicine, myfortic. And just as the incidences of actinic keratosis were reduced so were the problems of anal dysplasia.

I still am being followed carefully. Immune suppression is still an aspect of the drugs I'm taking for HIV and anti-rejection in relationship to my kidney transplant but the corner having been turned has made my life much easier.

Chapter 25

Esophageal Problems

And Lung Nodules

One of the drugs I had been prescribed along with the other anti-rejection drugs to protect my transplanted kidney was anti-gastric-esophageal-reflux medicine called omeprazole. This drug has been traditionally used for heartburn. At first it worked pretty well. A few months after the transplant, I was told to reduce the frequency of dosing from twice a day to once a day. When I reduced the frequency, I started to have a lot of heartburn.

My complaints about the pain resulted in the first of many endoscopies, upper GI scopes, to determine if there might be a tumor or some other growth in places like the esophagus. The first endoscopy performed by Dr. Schlager identified some polyps in my endoscopy but Dr. Schlager determined that it would be more dangerous to remove the polyps than to leave them in place.

He prescribed a medicine to alleviate my esophageal problems but the medicine interfered with the health of my transplanted kidney and therefore I had to stop taking it. Thus, the esophageal problems continued and I continued to complain, and then would be scheduled for more endoscopies. What happened more often than not is that when I went swimming and then ate my breakfast and took my medications, during the walk from the "Y" to the Embarcadero BART station, I would be in such extreme pain that I could barely move. After being seated on the train the pain subsided, but once I got off the train and walked to my bus stop the pain was just as bad as it had been before boarding the BART.

In 2015 when Steve and I went to New York and Washington for my nephew's graduation, I experienced one of the most painful episodes of esophageal pain. My primary physician, Dr. Hare, thought the culprit might simply be gas. When Steve and I visited him in May right after the graduation trip, Steve suggested that perhaps a CT scan would reveal a problem. Dr. Hare assented and I was scheduled very quickly for a CT scan.

The CT scan showed no problems with the esophagus, but there was something equally distressing. When the scan was read two small nodules in the lungs were revealed. They might portend something amiss, but they were not large enough to require anything more than a recheck CT scan in six months.

To be perfectly honest, I felt this was so inconsequential that it completely slipped my mind. So much, that when I was contacted in November 2015 that it was time for another CT scan, I asked why I did I need a CT scan? I was told and so it was scheduled.

CT scans are generally quite innocuous. They rarely take more than five minutes, where most of the time is spent removing overcoats and getting on the gurney that slides into the machine. One usually has to hold his breath three times, then it's over and the patient is on his way out.

But once this second CT scan was read, everything seemed to change. The November 2015 CT scan revealed that both the lung nodules discovered in May had grown. They had grown enough to set off some alarm bells. Dr. Hare called me to tell me that this result required more testing. A PET scan was ordered; it is much more complicated than a CT scan; it is longer in duration and also requires an injection of nuclear medicine in order to highlight problems in the possibly cancerous nodules, and oh yes, it is the first step in determining if a patient has cancer.

Now, having read this far, you are well aware that I have had an extremely complicated medical history, but for some reason or other, this hit me as hard as my AIDS diagnosis had in 1993. I was extremely frightened by the PET can and the possible side-effects of which I had read. Fortunately for me I had a friend, a former colleague of my father who had been battling lung cancer for many years. She had been subjected to many PET scans as well as radiation, chemotherapy and surgery. One of the qualities that had made her so attractive to me was her ability to maintain a cheery disposition in spite of all the medical challenges she had had to face.

As the fears and apprehensions about the PET scans grew more daunting, I realized that a quick phone call to my friend Barbara for reassurance was a possible solution. I called her several nights before the scan and she told me I would not encounter any difficulties. It might be long and uncomfortable, but it would not pose any problems. A huge weight was removed from my shoulders and I sailed through the PET scan without incident. Not only that, the scan, whose object was to highlight potential cancers, revealed nothing.

The next inquiry was set for March of 2016, and I could rest easy for the next three months. But this procedure had done nothing to improve my esophageal reflex problems. I resumed using the viscous lidocaine Dr. Hare had prescribed whenever I had a particularly annoying attack and we all went back to wondering why I was having so much trouble with heartburn, or esophageal reflux disease, or gas or whatever condition that was causing me so much pain.

Around the same time I started to have throbbing pain in the big toe of my left foot. That will be the subject of the next chapter.

Chapter 26

Dr. Chen

And

My Piscean Foot

In the Medieval Period it had become customary to divide the human body by the twelve signs of the Zodiac. This meant that a person's propensity to certain particular illnesses was governed by the sign of the Zodiac under which the person was born. Someone born at the beginning of the year (spring) in late March, which coincided with Gabriel's announcement to the Virgin Mary of the Savior's immanent birth, that person was born under the very first sign of the Zodiac, Aries. This sign governed any illness of the head. These governances proceeded in order from head to foot. And the last or twelfth sign governed the feet. So for persons born from February 21st to March 20th, their sign was Pisces and their principal medical difficulties were with their feet.

I was born on February 23rd, so it may comes as no surprise that I am particularly afflicted with many foot and toe problems. These problems occurred long before I became a Kaiser patient or was diagnosed with AIDS.

At the very beginning of my AIDS journey, I spent many unpleasant emergency appointments in the injury clinic with excruciatingly painful ingrown toe nails. But things got a lot worse with my feet and toes after my 2008 stroke. At first I developed plantar fasciitis. A podiatrist in the Injury clinic showed me some exercises and those pretty much took care of those painful problems.

But gradually, the bad habits I had developed after my stroke rehabilitation in Vallejo and the reliance on a very destructive manner of walking led to even more foot problems. One of the consequences of my left brain right sided stroke is that my right foot was altered so the foot was turned about 30^0. This turn required me to get orthotics that corrected the balance of my foot in a shoe. But there was an unanticipated problem that was a consequence of this condition. As the foot turned, the toes turned independently. When wearing socks with a sewn ridge next to the small toe, the toe that was no longer striking on the bottom or meaty part of the toe was now striking on the much less meaty side of the toe. This resulted in the continuous build-up of callouses. When I tried to remove these callouses by myself they frequently became infected and were very painful. One day I happened to have appointments with my three principal doctors: Dr. Follansbee, Dr. Goldstein and Dr. Yankulin. All three said that they could not see anything wrong, but Dr. Yankulin referred me to a Kaiser podiatrist, Dr. Chen, but the Mother's Day weekend of 2013 intervened, and I spent the most miserable Mother's Day weekend I can remember. When I finally was able to be seen by Dr. Chen at the beginning of the week, her expert eyes immediately identified an inflamed infection. She did a very painful clean-up of my infected toe and sent me home to a long convalescence.

At first, I doubted whether Dr. Chen would become one of my favorite providers, but through dogged friendly diligence she nursed me back to full use of my feet, and every time I saw her I felt better and better.

Eventually she sent me to get new orthotics, better socks and brand new seamless shoes. It didn't mean all my foot problems were solved, but at least I now had someone I trusted who knew how to deal with my foot and toe problems.

The next disaster she got to fix for me was the one I had caused by trying to trim my nails. Instead of trimming the nail I caused the toe to bleed and this resulted in another bad infection. This toe was on my left foot. This one had not been affected by my stroke. This problem was a direct result of my awkward trimming of a toe-nail on a toe twisted from the hereditary predisposition of a hammertoe. The infection and the subsequent surgical procedure occurred on Halloween 2014 the day of the Giant's World Series Victory Parade. The crowds were so thick and the street closures so onerous that I had a much more challenging walk to BART than I would have had had there been no parade.

Then in 2015, while I was dealing with lung nodules, and esophageal pain, the large toe of my left foot started to throb unceasingly. My first thought was an infection. I immediately sought Dr. Chen's care. But it wasn't infected. Instead it was determined by Drs. Chen, Yankulin, and Hare that I had gout.

One more malign condition, I thought. I was not drinking a sufficient amount of water and the cyclosporine that I had been taking to protect my kidney for the past six years had caused an increase in the levels of uric acid, thus precipitating the crystals that cause gout pain. Once it was explained to me by Drs. Yankulin and Chen, it made perfect sense. I would have to alter my already meagre diet. The good news was that what I thought was infected was not. The bad news was, as Dr. Yankulin always referred to each new diagnosis, another flower had joined my bouquet of illnesses.

Chapter 27

The Inevitable

Retirements

There is a challenge most of us never expect to face. When we are lucky enough to have medical professionals who are of similar ages to us, we never think about them retiring. Now it's not as though none of my prior doctors had retired before, but they generally were replaced by doctors I liked. But when I turned 60, in 2012, the first of my favorites, Dr. Rick Wolitz, who was a month older than I, decided he had had enough. His replacement was a very young woman named Dr. Isabella Phan. I was skeptical at first, but she eventually won my confidence. We would never have the kind of relationship I had had with Dr. Wolitz, however. He dragged me through the nightmare of CMV retinitis when that disease was a death sentence. There were no effective treatments but he tried everything. When the protease inhibitors were combined with other anti-retroviral medications, my T-cells rose and CMV retinitis was no longer a threat he still checked my vision and the progression of my disease but I only had to see him one every six months instead of once a week.

Shortly after my transition to Dr. Phan, I was having many new problems with my vision. My first concern was a resurgence of CMV retinitis, but this seemed highly unlikely since my T-cells were now in the high end of normal, and CMV only flourished when a patient's T-cells were below 100.

I scheduled an appointment with Dr. Phan and she quickly determined that I had significant cataracts in both of my eyes. Since I was nervous about any kind of surgery, I decided that my left eye should be done first. The first operation was in October, I wanted to wait until after Christmas to have the right eye done. I did not want my second surgery to impact our Christmas plans. But one of the problems I had not considered is that a new set of eyeglasses would not even be considered until both eyes had been changed. This created the expected but unconsidered problem that the glasses that had corrected the vision in both eyes would now only work for the uncorrected eye. And my mistake became obvious immediately after the first surgery.

I confessed my mistake to Dr. Phan and she told me that the only opportunity to address the other eye sooner would be only if another patient cancelled his or her surgery. Wonder of wonders, another patient cancelled and my right eye received its operation three weeks after the first.

Then the next problem occurred, I could not be examined for new glasses until a month after the second surgery. I scheduled my optometry for the date one month after the second surgery but there still was the matter of the glasses taking time to be produced.

I had decided that my distance vision had been corrected enough that I would not need lenses for distance. I thought I would only need the lenses for reading. Another big mistake; there is a distance for shopping and computer reading and the new reading glasses accommodated neither. Additionally, a place where I always need vision correction was for reading signs in museums.

Steve and I had two vacations planned to places with lots of museums, and if I did not get the new correction I needed, I would only be able to read and see distances, I would essentially be blind when it came to shopping, computers and museums, so I had to get my optometrist to give me an appropriate prescription for glasses that would address all my vision needs. Dr. Azus, the optometrist who has been taking care of my eyewear needs has been the incredibly friendly and efficient.

In 2013, while I was caring for my dying mother, I received a voice message from one of my other favorites. Dr. Goldstein, my dermatologist, who was also born in 1952, but where Dr. Wolitz was one month older than me, Dr. Goldstein was three months younger. His voice message actually brought tears to my eyes. He began it by saying that I was one of his favorite patients. Then he dropped the bomb. He had been fretting over how an early retirement would impact his most vulnerable patients, those like me who had been protected by his thorough and painstaking care. He had made sure that I had an appointment with him every month since my kidney transplant in July 2009.

When he told me that he had finally made the decision to retire for health reasons, it broke my heart. This most ardent advocate of my needs had decided to leave Kaiser and me. I was in shock. He had been a fighter in each dilemma I had faced over the past twenty years. When I needed approval for an insulin pump, he didn't rest a minute until it was approved. I remember Barbara Green, my diabetic nurse educator, asking me, "Why is your dermatologist, Sandy Goldstein, advocating for approval of an insulin pump for you?" I answered, "I don't know, I guess he just really is concerned about my health problems." When I was embroiled in the law suit with USAA over the car accident, he did everything possible to assist me. When I was posed with the prospect of losing the man who seemed to be my most important ally in any healthcare battle I faced at Kaiser, I went into shock. Fortunately, I was transitioned to Dr. Zipperstein who was Dr. Goldstein's own dermatologist.

After sixteen years of having Dr. Follansbee as my primary care provider, he told me in late 2013 that he planned to retire on February 28, 2014. He liked the numeric symmetry of that date. As he approached the date he felt that his replacement, Dr. Brad Hare, would be the most appropriate physician for me. I appreciated his advice and have had very good experiences with the man who was born the year I graduated from high school.

There were two more retiring medical professionals who were not doctors, they both were Diabetic Nurse Educators. The one who retired first was Barbara Green. She had been the person who had convinced me to use an insulin pump. She had been able to turn around my dreadful diabetic numbers. The excellent job she did for me got her a performance award and a raise in salary as she approached retirement. I was sad when I lost Barbara, but she was replaced by a wonderful new DNE, Nugget Burkhardt. Before I was sent to Barbara and Nugget, I had always viewed appointments with Diabetic Nurse Educators as the equivalent of a student being sent to the Dean's Office for disciplinary action. With Barbara and Nugget, I always felt I was visiting a friend who did not want to scold me but only to help me on a path to better sugar control. When each retired, it put me in another dilemma. Fortunately, Nugget was replaced with Phyllis who has been very helpful.

Then there was the bizarre and sudden departure of Dr. Joe Long. He had been treating my aggressive anal dysplasia. At first I was uncomfortable with his strange way of speaking. But as time went on he became a very comforting provider. He respected the fact that I could not tolerate his initially aggressive treatment, and adjusted his method to my sensibilities. Then in May 2015, just before my upcoming appointment I received an e-mail telling me that an upcoming appointment was being cancelled and the scheduler had no idea when a new surgeon would be in place. His sudden and mysterious disappearance to this day remains undisclosed and unexplained to me. Is his disappearance going to be explained when the details of the Kennedy assassination are fully revealed?

As the months went on, I finally asked Dr. Hare when this dangerous issue was going to be addressed. He said they were having trouble finding a replacement, and if I wanted to, I could be treated by the Nurse Practitioner in Oakland who was treating patients in a condition similar to mine. I decided to see the Oakland NP, Greg, and he treated me. I liked him, so I made the transition and it has worked out very well.

Chapter 28

The Unexpected

Disaster of

February 3, 2016

Prior to the weekend of January 30th and January 31st, I had had appointments with my primary care physician, Dr. Hare, and my dermatologist, Dr. Zipperstein. Both appointments had gone well for the first time in a long time. Neither physician proposed anything like surgery or biopsies. Dr. Hare knew I was concerned about the PET scan in December, but he expressed no alarm. He simply stated that I would require another CT scan in March, which at that time seemed far away. Dr. Zipperstein asked me to apply a cream to a basal cell cancer on my shin, but said no surgery would be necessary. I left both appointments very happy.

On Sunday Steve and I celebrated Bo's 11th birthday, which is the equivalent of 82 human years. Our previous dogs had died at 8 and 10, so we were very happy and grateful; Bo was young acting and still quite active; frequently acting like a puppy.

February started on Monday and Steve and I did our normal week day stuff; he went to his gym and I went to mine. I had no medical appointments until Thursday.

When I got up on Wednesday, February 3rd, I was awakened by the alarm at 5:30 AM. I got up, did my normal medical checks of weight, blood sugar, and blood pressure. I logged onto the internet and sent my usual e-mails and then got dressed. I did about twenty minutes of Kindle reading, went to the bedroom to say goodbye to Steve and Bo, then grabbed my lunch and my gym bag and headed out the door to catch the P bus, the Transbay bus that would take me from my Oakland home to the Embarcadero YMCA. I prefer the San Francisco Y to Oakland's because the pool is warmer and the workout rooms more conducive to the kinds of exercise I need to do.

Our four story condo building has a short sloped walkway which leads to a somewhat out of plum stairway at the top of which is covered entryway. As I exited the building I saw a bunch of newspapers thrown in a bunch on the slanted walkway. I knew Steve had subscribed to an abbreviated delivery of *The San Francisco Chronicle*. The delivery dates were Friday, Saturday and Sunday. Since this was a Wednesday, none of the papers in the bunch could be his. When Steve's papers were left on the walkway like these were, they were stolen, so I decided to be a Good Samaritan, I went down the steps and reached for the newspapers. I turned to throw them up on the porch in front of the door. The toss ended up forcing me to rely on my stroke-weakened right side and I lost my balance, I grabbed the nearest thing to my stroke-weakened right hand, a very fluid filled impatiens branch, this flimsy branch could not stabilize me and I very slowly fell to the stone filled concrete below me.

Immediately I knew something terrible had happened. I was able to roll away from resting on my painful right hip onto my left side. I actually thought for a brief moment that I would be able to rise from my fall and proceed to the bus stop to catch my Transbay San Francisco bound bus. But the second I tried to move anything I knew I was not going anywhere.

As I was falling a woman had been walking past me and she witnessed the entire fall. She immediately approached me and asked if she could do anything for me. I asked her if she could call my spouse whom I had just left. She told me that she did not have a cell phone. I asked her to reach into the left pocket of my jacket to get my phone. Since I had Steve's cell phone on my #2 speed-dial I told her to press and hold 2 to reach Steve. She did and she explained to Steve that I had had a dreadful fall and was writhing in pain in front of the building. Steve arrived in record time and on arrival dialed 911.

Then we waited for the Fire Department and ambulance to arrive. The seconds passed like hours. Finally, when both teams arrived, they proceeded with dispatch. The first thing they wanted to do was to remove my coat and pants. At first they planned to cut my clothes. I begged them not to do that.

With unbearable pain, I endured the removal of my North Face parka, my shoes and the Levi's I was wearing. I was in agony and virtually naked from the waist down, something I had not experienced prior to February 3, 2016.

The next thing that happened was that the EMT's rolled me onto a board and then shifted me onto the gurney that was immediately loaded into the ambulance. Then the questions began.

I noticed that the guy asking the questions was the younger of the two men who were assisting me. He would ask questions and then imply that he was checking his questions with the older guy. I began to feel like I was dealing with a rookie. The older guy said the younger guy needed to start an IV so they could start a flow of Fentanyl to minimize my pain. Surprisingly, despite his rookie status, he did an admirable job inserting the IV needle and beginning the Fentanyl flow.

The drive from our condo building to Kaiser is a little more than four blocks. Because of several less than satisfactory experiences at the old Oakland Kaiser Emergency Room and Hospital, I had usually been able to convince Steve to take me to San Francisco, rather than have an ambulance take the four blocks to Oakland's facility. But this time there was no chance of that happening. I could not even move and it took the professional men of the ambulance team to get me into the ambulance and drive me to the new Oakland Emergency Room and Hospital.

When one is wheeled on a gurney into an emergency room, it is like no other experience on earth. Simply being on an ambulance gurney does make one an object of fascination and pity. All the usual bureaucracy, delay and red tape experienced by an ambulatory emergency room patient were waived.

I was whisked past the receptionist and the nursing staff descended on me and proceeded to remove whatever clothes I was still wearing. They triaged me quickly and in a matter of minutes I was on my way to radiology. I asked for more fentanyl and was told that I would get something better, injectable dilaudid. There was the agonizing trip to get me to radiology and then the more excruciating slide onto the X-ray table.

Something completely new to me was the pneumatic pad on the bed that inflated to allow the nurses and technicians to more easily manipulate a patient. The first time this was done to me was when the personnel in radiology tried to move me to the very hard X-ray table. The inflation scared the daylights out of me. Then when they wanted to turn me on my side I practically fainted. They didn't and I was so grateful when the entire radiology experience was over.

Once I was wheeled back to the Emergency Room, the nurses inserted something called a nerve block. A needle was placed just above the fractured bone of my hip and a very strong anesthetic fluid was injected into my vein. In a short time it completely numbed my right leg, but it did absolutely nothing to arrest the pain in my fractured hip bone. The only medicine that had any effect on that pain was liquid dilaudid injected into my IV. But this miraculous medicine was only effective for about two hours, and then the pain was back just as bad as it had been after my fall.

While I was suffering from all this pain, Steve decided that he wanted to see Super Bowl City. Super Bowl 50 was going to be played in Santa Clara on Sunday, but San Francisco, former home of the 49ers, wanted some of those Super Bowl dollars, so SF was designated as the "host" city. Super Bowl City was a kind of circus that mainly served as a way of inconveniencing anyone who needed to be downtown but had little or no interest in the Super Bowl. Steve, as a long time 49er fan, wanted to see the circus, so he left me in the care of the nurses in the Emergency Room and took BART to San Francisco.

Meanwhile, I was waiting to be admitted and moved to a room in the hospital. Given the severity of my injury there were some medical providers who thought I would be in surgery that night. There were two obstacles blocking my path to surgery. One was directly related to my medications. The other was related to the Super Bowl. The medical problem was that since my stroke I had been taking a blood thinner called Aggrenox. Aggrenox was a red flag to the surgical team because of the bloodiness of the operation. The Super Bowl problem was more curious and insidious.

Apparently, big holidays and special events cause an unusual spike in freak accidents and automobile crashes, both of which have a deleterious impact on surgical operating rooms. Since Kaiser Oakland is recognized as one of the best trauma centers for orthopedic surgery in northern California, there were an inordinate number of critical cases that had inundated the Kaiser Oakland Surgery Department, and so injuries requiring surgery which were not life threatening were regarded as add-ons and therefore not very important.

So, under these circumstances, I was wheeled to my hospital room and told by my nurse on the 8th floor Orthopedic room that my surgery might be at any time. Despite the fact that I had had nothing to eat except for a couple of crackers given to me by the nursing staff in the Emergency Room before I was admitted to what would be my home prior to surgery and during my post-operative recuperation, eating was entirely out of the question.

Shortly after my arrival in my hospital room, my nurse told me that he would need to insert a catheter in my penis prior to what he said would be my immanent surgery. I was terrified of having another catheter inserted in my penis after the unfortunate two circumstances surrounding my kidney transplant operation. But this nurse was determined. Despite my fear and objections he got everything ready for the insertion including placing all the materials including the catheter on my bed next to my penis. But as he started to insert this diabolical device the pain he induced was unendurable and therefore he had to admit his failure and told me the operating staff would have to insert it after I had been anesthetized.

Steve arrived from his visit to Super Bowl City about the time that I was transferred from the Emergency Room to my north facing room on the 8th floor. Steve stayed for a little while but left before the trauma of the Foley catheter happened.

Then I was left alone expecting someone to come to get me and bring down to the basement where the operating rooms were located. I waited, and waited and waited. And then my nurse came in and told me the operation would not take place on February 3rd. We would begin the waiting period on Thursday, the following day. The nurse and everyone else suddenly wanted me to eat dinner and take my medications which had been delayed all day. I told them it was too late for either and I would not eat or take any medication until the next meal time. They shook their heads and left me alone. As usual I had a great deal of trouble getting any sleep in my hospital bed. I could not move my body because any movement of my body caused intolerable pain despite the IV dilaudid and the nerve block placed just above my fractured hip.

The next day started with the arrival of the phlebotomist before the sun rose. He was followed by the nurse's assistant who took my vital signs, then the nurse arrived to tell me that I would not be allowed to have any food water or medicine because my surgery had been scheduled for an early morning appointment in the operating room.

As the morning progressed, I was still told that my surgery was immanent but an emergency case had bumped it. I was still not allowed to have anything by mouth, not necessary medicine, food or water. Since I was not getting any nourishment, the nurses had to keep checking my blood sugars every four hours because of my insulin pump.

Finally, in the middle of the afternoon, I called Steve and asked him to contact Dr. Yankulin by KP.org to inform him that I had not had any of my anti-rejection medicines or anything else for two days. I figured if anyone could get things moving, he could.

The day ended without any news about surgery. About 11 PM, the nurses said that since I was not going to have my surgery until at least the following morning, would I be willing to eat something and take some of my medicines? I gave them an emphatic "NO!" and tried to get some sleep in my state of near starvation.

I'm not sure what Dr. Yankulin did, but the next day after the usual medical interruptions, I was told that my surgery would probably take place somewhere around noon, but I had been given permission to eat some breakfast and take my morning meds. The last time I had eaten or taken medicines was Tuesday night. At the time I was allowed to eat my Rice Krispies and toast it was 7 AM Friday. It had been quite an unintentional fast.

Even though there had been a glimmer of hope when I ate my breakfast, by noon I had had enough. I laid down the law. NO ONE WAS TO BE ALLOWED TO SAY ANYTHING ABOUT AN APPROACHING SURGERY. The first notice of an impending surgery was to be the arrival of the orderlies to escort my bed to the preparation area outside the Operating Room.

Finally, after agonizing days of painful waiting, the escorts arrived to take my bed and me to the basement where the operating rooms were located. When I arrived there, I was so relieved that the desperately necessary surgery was immanent, thus I was in a very good mood. There was an elaborate prep before the surgery. The litany of the medicines I was taking, and my medical history occupied a great deal of time. Fortunately, the nurse completing this process was very friendly, but there still were a couple of snags. Something that I needed for surgery, I forget what, was not immediately available and someone had to be dispatched to get it.

Then after two hours of preparation, I was wheeled into the Operating Room. Dr. Wang came in and introduced himself as the surgeon who was going to be the primary physician performing the operation. The anesthesiologist approached me and described what she was going to be using to anesthetize me. There was the usual identification roll call which had become very familiar to me throughout my many other surgeries. The drugs were allowed to enter my system, and I remember nothing else until I gradually resumed consciousness and I asked what the time was. It was 10:30 PM. I had been gone from my hospital room for four and a half hours.

Steve was in my room to greet me. The attendants in the Operating Room had called him when I had regained consciousness after my operation. It was wonderful to see him after my overly long awaited surgery. We both breathed a sigh of relief, but knew that the long road to recovery stretched out in front of us.

The following day, Saturday, February 6th, was a day packed with activity. I had a visit from my cousin Veronica who brought me some tulips. The first physical therapy round occurred when the therapist was able to actually get me out of bed and had me stand on my feet. It was very painful and extremely frightening. Another visitor was the Discharge Planner who was already discussing where I would be going once discharged. Depending on the speed of my recovery, the planner suggested the options were a skilled nursing facility or home. In the afternoon I saw three of my sponsees. Then in the evening my sister and brother-in-law visited. Over the past twenty-three years they had had an almost perfect record of visiting me when I had been hospitalized.

Steve brought a special Mardi Gras desert for us to share, the New Orleans treat originally from France, called "King Cake." The Carnival Season traditionally runs from Epiphany, the feast of the Three Kings visiting the infant Jesus, to Mardi Gras, the day before Ash Wednesday, the beginning of the fasting period of Lent. The cake itself is delicious and it was a great distraction to the real reason we were all gathered in my hospital room.

The next day, Sunday, February 7, 2016 was the long awaited and over hyped Super Bowl, one of the causes of the delay of my surgery. It was an extremely boring day for me. I did have an opportunity to take a short walk with my walker and one of the nurses' aides. Walking was still very painful and exhausting for me but I was grateful for the opportunity.

On Monday, it seemed that everything surrounding my care and future headed into high gear. The biggest issue was whether I would be heading home to receive in home rehabilitation, or sent to what was being referred to as a "Sniff," a code word for a Skilled Nursing Facility. Steve felt that Kaiser was trying to "dump" me on the street long before I was ready. Since the following day, Tuesday, which was also Mardi Gras and the New Hampshire Primary, was the day on which I was supposed to be released, the whole question of where I was going assumed much greater importance.

During my stay in Kaiser, the doctor who oversaw my continuing medical care, apart from my orthopedic care, was a hospitalist named Dr. Veejay. She was a native of India, and she was like no other doctor I had ever met. When she looked at me or at anyone, her concentration was amazing. It was as though she looked at my very soul. For the first three days, Wednesday, Thursday and Friday, I had not been able to take any drugs, so my difficulty with them was not an issue. But once Saturday dawned I explained to Dr. Veejay that I had been suffering from extreme esophageal reflux problems when I tried to swallow my very large pills. She didn't do what most other doctors had done, she didn't say there was nothing she could do about these problems, and instead she went straight to work and discovered that a number of these pills could be split. What a wonderful relief. For the first time someone had actually done something to address my problems with the pills.

I always enjoyed her visits and I felt she really had my best interest at heart.

It was because of these pills, or so I thought, that around 2 AM on the morning of Mardi Gras, Tuesday, February 9th, the day I thought I might be released from the hospital, I experienced extraordinary pain in the middle of my chest. It reminded me of every other gastro-esophageal pain I had experienced so I hit the nurse call button, and when she came I asked for the usual pain medicine I had been getting, IV dilaudid. This medicine was incredibly quick acting and I was asleep in no time.

I was awakened, as usual, by the phlebotomist making his morning blood draw. Shortly after I had my breakfast with my usual medicines and then saw Dr. Veejay and the orthopedic physician's assistant, Doug. Dr. Veejay was concerned about my pallor. She asked me what had happened during the night and I told her about my chest pain and the dilaudid.

Doug, the physician's assistant from orthopedics, discovered an unexpected leak from my surgical wound and arranged for a wound vacuum to be attached to my wound site and Dr. Veejay called for some special blood tests. At the time I thought it was just routine blood work. She didn't tell me that she had ordered the blood tests "stat," a medical term that means immediate. When she returned with the results, she informed that my troponin levels were very elevated. I had never heard of "troponin levels." I was informed that a normal troponin level was around .03, virtually a trace amount. My troponin level was 1.11. Then I was informed that a high troponin level indicated that a heart attack had happened. I was in shock and apparently very pale.

Dr. Veejay immediately ordered another IV in my arm and then started an IV of heparin to thin my blood. The reason for the second IV is that heparin cannot be mixed with any other drug, so in order to receive any other IV medication, it would have to be fed through the new IV. Then she ordered a telemetry monitor and told me that I was going to be moved from the orthopedic 8th floor to the telemetry 9th floor. But because there were no available beds on the 9th floor, a telemetry nurse had to baby sit me with a telemetry monitor while we waited for a 9th floor vacant room to become available.

Before I continue with my saga of a hip fracture hospitalization, I must account for the reason my unexpected heart attacks probably happened, it was not just a freak occurrence. There was a totally rational explanation for the heart attacks. In the autumn, in an effort to diminish my problems with esophageal reflux disease, Dr. Schlager suggested I stop taking baby aspirin. After trying every single statin on the market I had found that I had an allergic reaction to every single one. Then there was the very big problem. After my stroke, the stroke prevention medicine prescribed was a blood thinner aspirin-like drug called Aggrenox. Well, Aggrenox is usually stopped a week before surgery to prevent excessive bleeding. So the combination of all the risk factors plus the trauma of the fracture and the surgery to be performed in the absence of some drugs and the presence of others, created a perfect storm for heart attacks.

Sometime in the late afternoon, the bed movers arrived and took me and my bed up to the 9th floor. Unlike my room on the 8th floor which had a north view of Berkeley, the Richmond Bridge and Mount Tamalpais, my new room on the 9th floor faced south, with a view of Oakland, and our condo building. When Steve got home that evening after seeing me settled in my new 9th floor room, he called to tell me he was home. I told him I had been able to spot our condo from my room. I asked him to get the flashlight and I signaled him by turning my room light on and off and asked him to do the same with the flashlight. Since we watched the new Kaiser Hospital building being built and were disgusted by the way it had obscured our view of Mount Tamalpais, we knew we would be able to see the hospital from our balcony. We knew our building would be visible from the hospital, which part would be visible was the big question. Our building is nestled among many other mid-sized buildings and therefore only the top floor of our building is visible from Kaiser Hospital, which is where our penthouse is located. Only the very top of our building, our unit, is visible from the 9th floor and vice versa.

Well, so much about the location of my new room, now I must tell you about the big changes the move wrought. The main reason why the change had been made was because of my heart attacks and the need to have me on a floor with continuous telemetry monitoring. The previous floor had housed only orthopedic patients. The 9th Floor was predominantly telemetry monitored patients. As a result, the staff was very well acquainted with stroke and heart patients, but relatively unaware of the needs of patients like me who required rehabilitation after a disabling bone fracture.

At first I seemed to be getting along fine with the nurses on the 9th floor. I felt that the first nurse who cared for me was tremendously competent and responded with alacrity. When it was meal time, she knew that since I am a diabetic and she would need to be ready with the glucometer and my medications so that I could have them with my meal. She made sure I got my regular sessions of therapy and arranged for one of her nurse's aides to walk with me as was required as my rehabilitation. But when she was not there it seemed that no one else could do the job.

There was one particular night when my dinner was late in arriving, my medications were also late and when I asked if I could have my blood sugar tested so I could give myself the proper amount of insulin, she first looked at me as though I had lost my mind and then told me, with a straight face, that there were no orders for me either to be tested or dosed with insulin. She left to check if my request was legitimate and did not return for half an hour at which point my meal had become inedible. At that point I was so ready to be discharged from the hospital; I was at the point of making a break.

But it was not yet to be. Before I could be discharged I had to certify that I had recovered enough from my heart attacks that it was safe for me to go home and that the terms of my rehabilitation had been arranged. That involved Steve. The first issue decided was that although it might have been practical to send me to a Skilled Nursing Facility, the complicated regime regarding the dosing of my medications rendered that solution a non-starter. So the next complication was the hospital equipment that would be needed in our home. We have a two-story condominium and the bedroom is on a floor other than the main floor. I would need a hospital bed until I could take the stairs to the room with our bed. I would also need a commode over the toilet in order to use it safely. And I needed a walker. All these things had to be arranged through a Kaiser associate called Apria Healthcare.

Then there was the whole matter of post hospital rehabilitation. As long as I was confined to the house I would have to be checked by a visiting nurse who would also draw my blood. And this same Kaiser affiliate would provide personnel to be my physical and occupational therapists.

Finally, on February 13th I was released. My IV's were removed. I had my final consult with someone from the orthopedic department and a cardiologist. I was given my first set of post hospital appointments. I was allowed to get dressed and Steve went to bring the car to the wheel chair entrance of the hospital, and all I had to do was to sit and wait for the person who would push my wheelchair to the loading zone.

Our return to Oakland Avenue was amazing, the last time I had seen our condominium building it was through the back window of the ambulance that was taking me to Kaiser. On the journey home I was back in our car, facing the street ahead being driven home by Steve. It reminded me of those other journeys home after my stroke, my rehabilitation in Vallejo, my kidney transplant at UCSF, and my struggling walk after the Emergency Room experience that followed the car accident. As usual on my returns in a frail post-operative state, Steve had sequestered Bo in the TV room until I could get settled so that Bo would not overwhelm me.

The first thing I saw upon entrance was the hospital bed in the place in the living room which was usually occupied by the coffee table. Once I was seated, Steve allowed Bo to come out and greet me. I was so glad to see him and it reminded of the returns that had followed the other lengthy hospital stays.

One of the big changes I would have to face was bathing limitations. In our condo the upstairs bathroom has a typical bathroom/shower combination which was inaccessible to me as long as I had such limited use of my right leg while my hip was still so far from functioning normally. The downstairs bathroom had an unobstructed walk-in shower, but I had no idea when I would able to use the stairs.

Saturday was a very disorienting day but I was very glad to be home and out of the hospital. After we ate dinner Steve was able to get me settled in the study in my comfortable chair. I was so glad to be back to my DVD collection and the array of channels that were available on our cable fed televisions. I was also exhausted. Steve had thought of everything. I was able to move around with my walker, but every time I wanted to sit down, Steve had to move one of the dining room end chairs so that I could sit at the kitchen table or at the computer or anywhere else with the exception of my TV chair.

One of things we had to do before we went to bed on Saturday night was to fill my drug tray. There had been so many changes in my medications that the previously filled tray was no longer useful. I was so exhausted that Steve had to do most of the work.

When we woke up on Sunday morning, I was in my hospital bed and Steve had slept on the sofa in case any problems arose in the night. We had our usual breakfast and then Steve and Bo left for Point Isabel and Costco and I sat in the study and watched DVDs.

I was still having a lot of trouble with pain management and even though I had asked for dilaudid tablets I had been given Norco, which I hated. I tried to use Tylenol, but it simply was not strong enough. Sunday was a rather dismal day for me, but since the popular PBS television show *Downton Abbey*, which was in its final season, was on that night, Steve brought the dining room end chair into the TV room and I was able to watch the show with him.

Unfortunately, the TV show was interrupted by a very important phone call. The visiting nurse who wanted to come and enroll me in the care program she represented, do my vital signs and draw my blood, wanted to visit us on Monday. Although the phone call was an interruption, it was very important and settled a lot of questions.

The next day the enrollment happened and my physical therapist and the occupational therapist were assigned. My nurse turned out to be a very upbeat man named Julius, like many Filipino Americans, named for a very famous person from history, Julius Caesar. My physical therapist, whose initials mimicked his profession, PT, was named Peter. And my occupational therapist was a Los Angeles native named Eddie. I grew to like and appreciate them very much. They visited me about twice a week. Julius continued to monitor my vital signs and draw my blood. Peter started a very spirited course of exercises and Eddie assessed the challenges of getting dressed, getting in the shower, and getting into bed. Both of the therapists suggested items that could be purchased on Amazon.com.

At Costco Steve had seen a type of walker, which could also be used as a seat. He immediately suggested it; for one thing, it would alleviate the necessity of constantly moving one of the dining table chairs to wherever I needed to sit. I was hesitant to do anything that wasn't completely by the book. So, the first thing we asked Peter was what he thought of the Rollator. He recommended it enthusiastically and so I immediately purchased it.

As soon as we finished discussing the purchase of the Rollator, Peter said, "OK, we're going to do the stairs." This was not a question, but simply a statement of fact. I was hoping to postpone this part of my rehabilitation, but Peter knew if I was going to be able to take a shower, get rid of the hospital bed, and be able to sleep in our bed in the bedroom, I had to master the stairs. This would not only benefit me, but Steve as well. The reason being is that our couch was not comfortable and this would allow him to sleep downstairs too.

It was Peter's matter-of-fact way of introducing exercises and not questioning whether I was willing or able to do the exercises that increased his value as a therapist. We worked well together and I appreciated the challenges and his approval.

The same thing was true of Eddie, the occupational therapist. His focus was on personal care issues like dressing, showering, and getting into bed. He showed me tricks and utilitarian devices. He advocated a safer shower chair, a step aerobics platform to assist me in getting into our higher than normal bed, and a special bed side frame which I could use to pivot in and out of bed. The tools he suggested for my dressing needs were not practical for me to use.

Caesar the nurse, Peter the physical therapist, and Eddie the occupational therapist all finished the in-home care about three weeks after my return home. I was sad to see them end their service, but it did mean that I was getting better and able to return to out-patient care.

I will summarize this whole episode of my fractured hip and subsequent surgery, heart attacks, and home rehabilitation with a grateful salute to my spouse. Without question Steve went far beyond the call of duty. With the extreme disability that I now had to face, I could almost do nothing, even down to the simple rudiments of getting dressed. As long as I was unable to go downstairs where our bed and the walk-in shower were, Steve had to sleep upstairs on the couch in case I had some problem in the night. Before my fall, I had been responsible for one of Bo's daily walks and for the maintenance of our rooftop garden. After the accident I could do neither of these tasks and so Steve had to do all of these things. Saturday had been the day on which both of us split the house cleaning chores. Now Steve had to handle everything. In short he has been burning the candle at both ends and for the most part, with a smile on his face. Believe me; I have been very fortunate and blessed in the wonderful man who is my spouse. Without him this would have been an even more traumatic challenge, I am not sure I would have made it.

Chapter 29

Therapy After

The Hip Fracture

And

My Other

Therapeutic Care

At Kaiser

As you undoubtedly remember having read this book so far, you know that the therapy that I have received since my hip fracture is not my first encounter with Kaiser's Outpatient Physical Therapy Department. After my stroke in 2008 I was sent to Kaiser Foundation Rehabilitation Center, abbreviated KFRC, which were the call letters of a radio station which was the most popular station for the teens of the time when I was a teen and of my early adulthood. I felt that I was released from KFRC way too early, before I was ready.

Once I graduated from KFRC, I was sent to Kaiser Oakland's outpatient Physical Therapy Department. I was not very happy with my experience with the Oakland Therapists. They had not dealt with my challenges, the principal of them being my difficulty with walking. I had developed some inappropriate ways of moving my right foot which resulted in the destruction of all my right shoes.

Dissatisfied with what had happened at KFRC and Oakland Kaiser in regard to the rehabilitation of my right arm and hand, I asked to be transferred to San Francisco's Occupational Therapy.

In 2010 I was involved as a passenger in a car accident. The damage done to me was the breaking of three fingers of my previously damaged right hand. Since my right side was severely affected by my 2008 stroke, the impact of the car accident retarded whatever progress I had made with the rehabilitation of my hand and arm. Once my hand had healed enough to be rehabilitated, I was assigned to a San Francisco therapist. The therapist assigned to me was adequate but had the personality of a goldfish. I can't remember why I stopped working with this therapist but I did.

In April 2014, I had a smaller stroke than the one I had had in 2008, but it did affect my ability to walk and so I got another therapist. This one was very nice but relatively ineffective. I went through the motions and she seemed to be happy with my progress so that therapy ended much the way the other ones did.

In late 2014, I began to have trouble with my right leg while swimming; it had been a form of physical therapy which had made a phenomenal effect on the rehabilitation of my posture. When I was swimming one day I noticed how much weaker right leg felt than it had, making me think that I had had another stroke. I spoke to Dr. Yankulin, and he recommended his favorite physical therapist, a man who had the same name as I did. That seemed like a good omen.

When I started with Frank, I was impressed with his manner which indicated to me that the success of my therapy was up to me. Every other therapist, and please excuse what you might find sexist, most were female therapists, did not take this attitude. They rather assumed more than fifty percent of the responsibility for my recovery, and instead of challenging me to do my part, they merely took pity on me. With Frank the tactic was to challenge me and to remind me that others were more willing to recover than I seemed to be.

The way in which he treated me at first was somewhat off putting. Since I had been relying on swimming for my principal form of exercise, I was merely paying lip-service to the exercises he had given me, and avoiding them rather than doing them. He basically reacted with indifference and suggested that I might not really want to do therapy.

Then something unexpected happened. A skin cancer surgery prevented me from swimming for three weeks which forced me to start putting a lot more energy into Frank's exercises. Gradually I began to notice significant changes in my gait, my walking was improving. My right leg was stronger and I saw that all the work that Frank had assigned me was really paying off.

Medicare has a limit on how much time and money can be spent on physical rehabilitation. By the time of my hip fracture I was approaching that limit. I had two more scheduled appointments with Frank and then it would be over. But the accident changed everything, I would be returning to Frank to continue my post hip surgery rehabilitation.

I need to say one more thing about physical therapy. Women have an edge in population numbers in relationship to men. I don't know what the therapist numbers are but because of the physical differences between men and women my experience is that men know better how to deal with disabilities of men and are more able to motivate men than women are. At least that has been my experience. I have had much better experiences with male therapists than with female therapists. My impression is that males know more about the movements and mechanics of the male body. Additionally, they tend to be more demanding of other males challenging us to do more than we think we can. With female therapists I was usually babied or mothered, neither method worked for me.

Chapter 30

The Rest of the Story

In this chapter I want to make my final remarks about the good and bad at Kaiser. With regard to the good it's very easy. The medical staff is incredible. I wouldn't be alive if it weren't. The place where the problem is most acute is with the support staff. The haphazard way in which they seem to be trained leads to a very distressing situation. Some of the receptionists and medical assistants behave as though the patients are doing them a favor by coming to Kaiser. This is also frequently true of the hospital nurses and the pharmacy clerks.

Phoning Kaiser can be tremendously exhausting as the caller is put through a labyrinthine phone tree, and then when one gets an actual human that human asks for all the information that has been given electronically to get to an actual human.

The worst example of this inefficiency is shown by the Durable Medical Equipment Department. Unlike the very efficient online pharmacy available through KP.org, the DME, which dispenses supplies which cannot be ordered through the pharmacy, uses an extremely frustrating, antediluvian and inefficient phone mail system. There is no record of the patient's call to which the patient can refer, so that the patient has no idea if the order has been filled or lost, until in some cases it is already too late to receive the order. Without question, this has been the most frequent cause of frustration for me at Kaiser.

Since these are my concluding remarks I can only say how grateful I am for having joined Kaiser almost thirty years ago, when I got my first benefits package when I worked at Industrial Indemnity. It was the cheapest option available to me back in 1987. At that time its reputation was lower than many of the private pay options. But when malpractice Insurance premiums skyrocketed, many excellent doctors who wished to receive a salary rather than have to pay for facilities, staff and their malpractice insurance, decided that working for a Health Maintenance Organization was a much better option for them, they joined Kaiser and its patients benefitted exponentially.

My Kaiser journey is not over thanks in no small part to the outstanding medical care I have received there. But this book is done.

www.ingramcontent.com/pod-product-compliance
Lightning Source LLC
Chambersburg PA
CBHW070221190526
45169CB00001B/39